KV-086-894

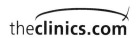
theclinics.com

CLINICS IN PERINATOLOGY

Cesarean Delivery: Its Impact on the Mother and Newborn, Part I

GUEST EDITORS
Lucky Jain, MD, MBA
Ronald Wapner, MD

June 2008 • Volume 35 • Number 2

SAUNDERS

An Imprint of Elsevier, Inc.
PHILADELPHIA   LONDON   TORONTO   MONTREAL   SYDNEY   TOKYO

W.B. SAUNDERS COMPANY
A Division of Elsevier Inc.

Elsevier, Inc., 1600 John F. Kennedy Blvd., Suite 1800, Philadelphia, PA 19103-2899

http://www.theclinics.com

CLINICS IN PERINATOLOGY	**Volume 35, Number 2**
June 2008	**ISSN 0095-5108**
Editor: Carla Holloway	**ISBN-10: 1-4160-5799-4**
	ISBN-13: 978-1-4160-5799-4

The ideas and opinions expressed in *Clinics in Perinatology* do not necessarily reflect those of the Publisher. The Publisher does not assume any responsibility for any injury and/or damage to persons or property arising out of or related to any use of the material contained in this periodical. The reader is advised to check the appropriate medical literature and the product information currently provided by the manufacturer of each drug to be administered, to verify the dosage, the method and duration of administration or contraindications. It is the responsibility of the treating physician or other health care professional, relying on independent experience and knowledge of the patient, to determine drug dosages and the best treatment for the patient. Mention of any product in this issue should not be construed as endorsement by the contributors, editors, or the Publisher of the product or manufacturers' claims.

Clinics in Perinatology (ISSN 0095-5108) is published in quarterly by Elsevier Inc., 360 Park Avenue South, New York, NY 10010-1710. Months of issue are March, June, September, and December. Business and Editorial offices: 1600 John F. Kennedy Blvd., Suite 1800, Philadelphia, PA 19103-2899. Customer Service Office: 6277 Sea Harbor Drive, Orlando, FL 32887-4800. Periodicals postage paid at New York, NY and additional mailing offices. Subscription prices are $197.00 per year (US individuals), $297.00 per year (US institutions), $232.00 per year (Canadian individuals), $369.00 per year (Canadian institutions), $268.00 per year (foreign individuals), $369.00 per year (foreign institutions) $95.00 per year (US students), and $131.00 per year (Canadian and foreign students). Foreign air speed delivery is included in all Clinics subscription prices. All prices are subject to change without notice. **POSTMASTER:** Send address changes to *Clinics in Perinatology*; Elsevier Periodicals Customer Service, 6277 Sea Harbor Drive, Orlando, FL 32887-4800. Customer Service: 1-800-654-2452 (US). From outside the United States, call 1-407-563-6020. Fax: 1-407-363-9661. E-mail: JournalsCustomerService-usa@elsevier.com.

Clinics in Perinatology is also pubilshed in Spanish by McGraw-Hill Interamericana Editores S.A., P.O. Box 5-237, 06500 Mexico D.F., Mexico.

Clinics in Perinatology is covered in *MEDLINE/PubMed (Index Medicus), Current Contents, Excepta Medica, BIOSIS* and *ISI/BIOMED.*

Printed in the United States of America.

GUEST EDITORS

LUCKY JAIN, MD, MBA, Richard W. Blumberg Professor; Executive Vice Chairman, Department of Pediatrics, Emory University School of Medicine, Atlanta, Georgia

RONALD WAPNER, MD, Professor; Director, Maternal Fetal Medicine, Department of Obstetrics and Gynecology, Columbia University School of Medicine, New York, New York

CONTRIBUTORS

IRA ADAMS-CHAPMAN, MD, Assistant Professor of Pediatrics; Director, Developmental Progress Clinic, Emory University School of Medicine, Atlanta, Georgia

VANI R. BETTEGOWDA, MHS, Perinatal Data Center, National Office, March of Dimes Foundation, White Plains, New York

WILLIAM M. CALLAGHAN, MD, MPH, Division of Reproductive Health, National Center for Chronic Disease Prevention and Health Promotion, Centers for Disease Control and Prevention, Atlanta, Georgia

KARLA DAMUS, RN, PhD, Department of Obstetrics, Gynecology, and Women's Health, Albert Einstein College of Medicine, Bronx, New York

MICHAEL J. DAVIDOFF, MPH, Perinatal Data Center, National Office, March of Dimes Foundation, White Plains, New York

EUGENE DECLERCQ, PhD, Department of Maternal and Child Health, Boston University School of Public Health, Boston, Massachusetts

TODD DIAS, MS, Perinatal Data Center, National Office, March of Dimes Foundation, White Plains, New York

SNEHAL DOSHI, MD, MSEd, Fellow, Department of Pediatrics; Division of Neonatology, University of Texas Medical Branch, Galveston, Texas

WILLIAM A. ENGLE, MD, Erik T. Ragan Professor of Pediatrics, Section of Neonatal-Perinatal Pediatrics, Indiana University School of Medicine, Indianapolis, Indiana

KARIN FUCHS, MD, Clinical Fellow, Division of Maternal Fetal Medicine, Columbia University Medical Center, New York, New York

CYNTHIA GYAMFI, MD, Assistant Clinical Professor, Division of Maternal Fetal Medicine, Columbia University Medical Center, New York, New York

SHANNON E.G. HAMRICK, MD, Department of Pediatrics, Emory University, Emory Children's Center, Atlanta, Georgia

LUCKY JAIN, MD, MBA, Richard W. Blumberg Professor; Executive Vice Chairman, Department of Pediatrics, Emory University School of Medicine, Atlanta, Georgia

MARK KLEBANOFF, MD, MPH, Division of Epidemiology, Statistics and Prevention Research, *Eunice Kennedy Shriver* National Institute of Child Health and Human Development, National Institutes of Health, Department of Health and Human Services, Bethesda, Maryland

MICHELLE A. KOMINIAREK, MD, Assistant Professor of Clinical Obstetrics and Gynecology, Division of Maternal Fetal Medicine, Indiana University School of Medicine, Indianapolis, Indiana

MARIAN F. MACDORMAN, PhD, Reproductive Statistics Branch, Division of Vital Statistics, National Center for Health Statistics, Centers for Disease Control and Prevention, Hyattsville, Maryland

MICHAEL H. MALLOY, MD, MS, Professor, Department of Pediatrics; Division of Neonatology, University of Texas Medical Branch, Galveston, Texas

FAY MENACKER, DrPH, CPNP, Reproductive Statistics Branch, Division of Vital Statistics, National Center for Health Statistics, Centers for Disease Control and Prevention, Hyattsville, Maryland

JOANN R. PETRINI, PhD, MPH, Perinatal Data Center, National Office, March of Dimes Foundation, White Plains; Department of Obstetrics, Gynecology, and Women's Health, Albert Einstein College of Medicine, Bronx, New York

ASHWIN RAMACHANDRAPPA, MD, MPH, Fellow, Division of Neonatology, Department of Pediatrics, Emory University School of Medicine, Atlanta, Georgia

DOLLY SHARMA, MD, Pediatric Infectious Diseases, Emory University School of Medicine, Atlanta, Georgia

CAROLINE SIGNORE, MD, MPH, Pregnancy and Perinatology Branch, *Eunice Kennedy Shriver* National Institute of Child Health and Human Development, National Institutes of Health, Department of Health and Human Services, Bethesda, Maryland

PAUL SPEARMAN, MD, Pediatric Infectious Diseases, Emory University School of Medicine, Atlanta, Georgia

HELEN O. WILLIAMS, MD, Assistant Professor, Department of Pediatrics, Emory University School of Medicine, Atlanta, Georgia

CONTRIBUTORS

CONTENTS

The percentage of United States cesarean births increased from
20.7% in 1996 to 31.1% in 2006. Cesarean rates increased for women
of all ages, race/ethnic groups, and gestational ages and in all
states. Both primary and repeat cesareans have increased. Increases
in primary cesareans in cases of "no indicated risk" have been
more rapid than in the overall population and seem the result of
changes in obstetric practice rather than changes in the medical risk
profile or increases in "maternal request." Several studies note an
increased risk for neonatal and maternal mortality for medically
elective cesareans compared with vaginal births.

The increasing trend of delivering at earlier gestational ages has
raised concerns of the impact on maternal and infant health. The
delicate balance of the risks and benefits associated with continuing a pregnancy versus delivering early remains challenging.
Among singleton live births in the United States, the proportion of
preterm births increased from 9.7% to 10.7% between 1996 and
2004. The increase in singleton preterm births occurred primarily
among those delivered by cesarean section, with the largest
percentage increase in late preterm births. For all maternal
racial/ethnic groups, singleton cesarean section rates increased
for each gestational age group. Singleton cesarean section rates for
non-Hispanic black women increased at a faster pace among all

preterm gestational age groups compared with non-Hispanic white and Hispanic women. Further research is needed to understand the underlying reasons for the increase in cesarean section deliveries resulting in preterm birth.

Late Preterm Infants, Early Term Infants, and Timing of Elective Deliveries

William A. Engle and Michelle A. Kominiarek

Delivery of infants who are physiologically mature and capable of successful transition to the extrauterine environment is an important priority for obstetric practitioner. A corollary of this goal is to avoid iatrogenic complications of prematurity and maternal complications from delivery. The purpose of this review is to describe the consequences of birth before physiologic maturity in late preterm and term infants, to identify factors contributing to the decline in gestational age of deliveries in the United States, and to describe strategies to reduce premature delivery of late preterm and early term infants.

The Influence of Obstetric Practices on Late Prematurity

Karin Fuchs and Cynthia Gyamfi

In this article, the authors review the standard management of several maternal and fetal complications of pregnancy and examine the effect these practices may have on the late preterm birth rate. Given the increasing rate of late preterm birth and the increased recognition of the morbidity and mortality associated with delivery between 34 and 37 weeks, standard obstetric practices and practice patterns leading to late preterm birth should be critically evaluated. The possibility of expectant management of some pregnancy complications in the late preterm period should be investigated. Furthermore, prospective research is warranted to investigate the role of antenatal corticosteroids beyond 34 weeks.

Neonatal Morbidity and Mortality After Elective Cesarean Delivery

Caroline Signore and Mark Klebanoff

This article explores the effects of elective cesarean delivery (ECD) at term on neonatal morbidity and mortality. Available data have limitations, and do not provide conclusive evidence regarding the safety of planned ECD versus planned vaginal delivery. Some data suggest an association between ECD and increased neonatal respiratory morbidity and lacerations, and possibly decreased central and peripheral nervous system injury. Potentially increased risks of neonatal mortality with ECD at term may be counterbalanced by risks for fetal demise in ongoing pregnancies. Patients and physicians considering ECD should review competing risks and benefits; further research is needed to inform these discussions.

Elective Cesarean Section: Its Impact on Neonatal Respiratory Outcome

Ashwin Ramachandrappa and Lucky Jain

Physiologic events in the last few weeks of pregnancy coupled with the onset of spontaneous labor are accompanied by changes in the hormonal milieu of the fetus and its mother, resulting in preparation of the fetus for neonatal transition. Rapid clearance of fetal lung fluid is a key part of these changes, and is mediated in large part by transepithelial sodium reabsorption through amiloride-sensitive sodium channels in the alveolar epithelial cells, with only a limited contribution from mechanical factors and Starling forces. This article discusses the respiratory morbidity associated with elective cesarean section, the physiologic mechanisms underlying fetal lung fluid absorption, and potential strategies for facilitating neonatal transition when infants are delivered by elective cesarean section before the onset of spontaneous labor.

Cesarean Delivery and Its Impact on the Anomalous Infant

Shannon E.G. Hamrick

Although cesarean deliveries frequently are performed for anomalous fetal conditions, available data do not always support a fetal benefit from this delivery management. The literature on cesarean delivery for anomalous infants reports insufficient information on comorbid neonatal conditions, so these complications are unknown in this population of newborns. In a minority of cases, a cesarean delivery is reasonable to prevent dystocia or optimize outcome. Areas for future investigation include prospective, randomized, controlled trials of prelabor cesarean compared with vaginal deliveries for myelomeningocele and anterior abdominal wall defects. The rarity of other lesions likely precludes randomized controlled trials.

The Impact of Cesarean Delivery on Transmission of Infectious Agents to the Neonate

Dolly Sharma and Paul Spearman

The rate of cesarean deliveries has increased dramatically over the past decade. Studies to date have highlighted a number of factors on the part of the treating physician and the expectant mother contributing to this increase. Maternal infections are not a major cause of this increase. There are a limited number of infections in a pregnant woman that warrant cesarean delivery to prevent perinatal transmission. This article outlines those infections known to be transmitted perinatally through the infected birth canal and details the current recommendations for cesarean delivery. Pregnant women with active genital herpes lesions or with known herpes simplex virus infection and a prodromal illness consistent with recurrence at the time of presentation in labor should undergo cesarean delivery. Pregnant women who are HIV infected and have detectable viremia (>1000 copies/mL) should be counseled regarding the potential benefits of cesarean delivery as an adjunct to antiretroviral therapy. Hepatitis C virus (HCV) can be transmitted intrapartum, but prevention of HCV transmission by cesarean delivery has not been proved effective and is not generally indicated. A limited number of other infectious agents can be transmitted through the birth canal but do not constitute an indication for cesarean delivery.

GOAL STATEMENT

The goal of *Clinics in Perinatology* is to keep practicing neonatologists and maternal-fetal medicine specialists up to date with current clinical practice in perinatology by providing timely articles reviewing the state of the art in patient care.

ACCREDITATION

The *Clinics in Perinatology* is planned and implemented in accordance with the Essential Areas and Policies of the Accreditation Council for Continuing Medical Education (ACCME) through the joint sponsorship of the University of Virginia School of Medicine and Elsevier. The University of Virginia School of Medicine is accredited by the ACCME to provide continuing medical education for physicians.

The University of Virginia School of Medicine designates this educational activity for a maximum of 60 *AMA PRA Category 1 Credits*™. Physicians should only claim credit commensurate with the extent of their participation in the activity.

The American Medical Association has determined that physicians not licensed in the US who participate in this CME activity are eligible for *AMA PRA Category 1 Credits*™.

Credit can be earned by reading the text material, taking the CME examination online at: http://www.theclinics.com/home/cme, and completing the evaluation. After taking the test, you will be required to review any and all incorrect answers. Following completion of the test and evaluation, your credit will be awarded and you may print your certificate.

FACULTY DISCLOSURE/CONFLICT OF INTEREST

The University of Virginia School of Medicine, as an ACCME accredited provider, endorses and strives to comply with the Accreditation Council for Continuing Medical Education (ACCME) Standards of Commercial Support, Commonwealth of Virginia statutes, University of Virginia policies and procedures, and associated federal and private regulations and guidelines on the need for disclosure and monitoring of proprietary and financial interests that may affect the scientific integrity and balance of content delivered in continuing medical education activities under our auspices.

The University of Virginia School of Medicine requires that all CME activities accredited through this institution be developed independently and be scientifically rigorous, balanced and objective in the presentation/discussion of its content, theories and practices.

All authors/editors participating in an accredited CME activity are expected to disclose to the readers relevant financial relationships with commercial entities occurring within the past 12 months (such as grants or research support, employee, consultant, stock holder, member of speakers bureau, etc.). The University of Virginia School of Medicine will employ appropriate mechanisms to resolve potential conflicts of interest to maintain the standards of fair and balanced education to the reader. Questions about specific strategies can be directed to the Office of Continuing Medical Education, University of Virginia School of Medicine, Charlottesville, Virginia.

The authors/editors listed below have identified no professional or financial affiliations for themselves or their spouse/partner:
Ira Adams-Chapman, MD; Vani R. Bettegowda, MHS; Robert Boyle, MD (Test Author); William M. Callaghan, MD, MPH; Karla Damus, RN, PhD; Michael J. Davidoff, MPH; Eugene Declercq, PhD; Todd Dias, MS; Snehal Doshi, MD, MSEd.; William A. Engle, MD; Karin M. Fuchs, MD; Cynthia Gyamfi, MD; Shannon E.G. Hamrick, MD; Carla Holloway (Acquisitions Editor); Mark Klebanoff, MD, MPH; Michelle A. Kominiarek, MD; Marian F. MacDorman, PhD; Michael H. Malloy, MD, MS; Fay Menacker, DrPH, CPNP; Joann R. Petrini, PhD, MPH; Ashwin Ramachandrappa, MD, MPH; Dolly Sharma, MD; Caroline Signore, MD, MPH; Paul Spearman, MD; Ronald Wapner, MD (Guest Editor); and Helen O. Williams, MD.

The authors/editors listed below identified the following professional or financial affiliations for themselves or their spouse/partner:
Lucky Jain, MD, MBA (Guest Editor) serves on the Speaker's bureau for IKARIA, and is an independent contractor for Schering Plough.

Disclosure of Discussion of non-FDA approved uses for pharmaceutical products and/or medical devices:
The University of Virginia School of Medicine, as an ACCME provider, requires that all faculty presenters identify and disclose any "off label" uses for pharmaceutical and medical device products. The University of Virginia School of Medicine recommends that each physician fully review all the available data on new products or procedures prior to instituting them with patients.

TO ENROLL

To enroll in the Clinics in Perinatology Continuing Medical Education program, call customer service at: 1-800-654-2452 or visit us online at: www.theclinics.com/home/cme. The CME program is available to subscribers for an additional fee of $195.00.

FORTHCOMING ISSUES

RECENT ISSUES

Preface

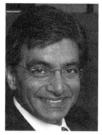 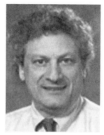

Lucky Jain, MD, MBA   Ronald Wapner, MD
Guest Editors

How will our grandchildren be delivered?

Who would have thought that we would be asking this question in the year 2008? Yet the current debate on the pros and cons of vaginal and cesarean births is more vociferous than ever, spurred, in particular, by the rapid rise in cesarean births. Rising from a mere 5% of total births in the United States in 1970, this year nearly one out of every three births in the United States will occur by operative delivery. The rate of rise is even more spectacular in some other countries. The highly publicized decisions by celebrities to have cesarean births and the lay information related to pelvic floor dysfunction, among other things, may be encouraging some mothers to recommend their own mode of delivery. This decade will go down in history as the decade when "cesarean delivery on maternal request" became an official term!

One wonders, though, why there is all this fuss over an aspect of human life that has coexisted in harmony with the medical profession for hundreds of years. There is evidence to show that cesarean births have improved the outcome in several high-risk categories, such as breech presentation, very early gestations, and in cases where there is evidence of fetal distress. However, new concerns have emerged about the short- and long-term risks and benefits of either mode of delivery. The absence of clear evidence to show that one is better than the other has led to a conundrum. As would be expected, maternal benefits are sometimes at odds with neonatal interests. There is fascinating anthropological information that shows the

0095-5108/08/$ - see front matter © 2008 Elsevier Inc. All rights reserved.
doi:10.1016/j.clp.2008.03.012

progressively increasing brain volume (eg, skull size) of the human fetus at birth, coupled with the concomitant changes in the pelvic anatomy as a result of bipedalism, may have set up a natural conflict for spontaneous vaginal birth for future generations.

So how do we resolve this issue and provide an evidence-based recommendation to families seeking counsel for one of the most important decisions of their reproductive lives? Some have suggested that a randomized head-to-head trial of low-risk or no-risk mothers comparing cesarean to vaginal birth is essential—perhaps the only definitive way to answer this question. However, cost and logistical issues notwithstanding, it is not clear how such a study could be pulled off, given the huge number of participants it would need and the ethical debate it would be certain to stir.

One good outcome of all this is the much needed attention this subject is finally receiving. This first-ever issue of the *Clinics in Perinatology* devoted to cesarean delivery is an example of that. We are particularly delighted to spearhead this two-issue offering of *Clinics in Perinatology* dedicated entirely to cesarean birth. The first issue focuses on the epidemiology and neonatal outcomes after cesarean section. The second issue, due to be published later this year, will focus on maternal topics. We are very grateful to Carla Holloway at Elsevier for her unwavering support, and to all of our colleagues who have contributed to this project.

We hope this compilation of articles by experts in the field will serve as a handy reference for a variety of topics related to cesarean birth. Meanwhile, the search for the ideal mode of delivery for the next generation and the next will continue!

Lucky Jain, MD, MBA
Department of Pediatrics
Emory University School of Medicine
2015 Uppergate Drive NE
Atlanta, GA 30322, USA

E-mail address: ljain@emory.edu

Ronald Wapner, MD
Maternal Fetal Medicine
Department of Obstetrics and Gynecology
Columbia University School of Medicine
New York, NY 10021, USA

E-mail address: Rw2191@columbia.edu

ELSEVIER
SAUNDERS

CLINICS IN
PERINATOLOGY

Clin Perinatol 35 (2008) 293–307

Cesarean Birth in the United States: Epidemiology, Trends, and Outcomes

Marian F. MacDorman, PhD[a],*, Fay Menacker, DrPH, CPNP[a], Eugene Declercq, PhD[b]

[a]Reproductive Statistics Branch, Division of Vital Statistics, National Center for Health Statistics, Centers for Disease Control and Prevention, 3311 Toledo Road, Room 7318, Hyattsville, MD 20782, USA
[b]Department of Maternal and Child Health, Boston University School of Public Health, 715 Albany Street, Boston, MA, USA

The percentage of all births in the United States that are cesarean deliveries has increased substantially in recent years, from 20.7% in 1996 to an all-time high of 31.1% in 2006 [1,2]. Cesarean delivery currently is the most common major surgical procedure for women in the United States [3] with more than 1.3 million cesareans performed annually [1]. The cesarean rate increased dramatically during the 1970s and early 1980s and began to decline in the late 1980s (based on data from the National Hospital Discharge Survey). Between 1989 and 1996 the total cesarean rate decreased as a result of a decrease in the primary rate and an increase in the rate of vaginal birth after cesarean (VBAC). Since 1996, these trends have reversed, and increases have been rapid and sustained for primary and repeat cesareans over the past decade [2]. This article examines recent trends in cesarean delivery for the overall population and for women who have no reported medical indications for cesarean delivery, and it examines neonatal outcomes for primary cesarean births among low-risk women.

Methods

Data on cesarean delivery used in this article are based on the method of delivery as reported on the more than 4 million birth certificates filed each

The findings and conclusions in this article are those of the authors and do not necessarily represent the views of the Centers for Disease Control and Prevention.

* Corresponding author.
  E-mail address: mfm1@cdc.gov (M.F. MacDorman).

year in the United States and compiled by the National Center for Health Statistics (NCHS). Cesarean data became available from birth certificates in 1989, and by 1991 all states and the District of Columbia were reporting this information. Before 1989, data from the National Hospital Discharge Survey were used to track trends in cesarean delivery.

Several measures of cesarean delivery are used and computed as follows. The total cesarean rate is the percent of cesarean births of all births in a given year. The primary rate is the percent of cesarean births among women in a given year who have not had a previous cesarean delivery. The rate of repeat cesarean delivery is the percent of all cesarean births among women who have had a previous cesarean. A related measure, the rate of VBAC, is defined as the percent of vaginal births among women who have had a previous cesarean.

This article examines changes in cesarean rates among all United States mothers by maternal age, race/ethnicity, gestational age, and state. Total cesarean rates are examined from 1989 to 2006 whereas primary and repeat cesarean rates are examined from 1989 to 2004. National estimates of primary and repeat cesarean rates for 2005 and 2006 are not available because of a change in the wording and formatting of the question on prior cesareans between the 1989 and the 2003 revisions of the United States Standard Certificate of Birth. Because of the staggered implementation of the 2003 revision among states, both revisions currently are in use in different states, making national estimates of primary and repeat cesareans problematic, although state-level estimates are available.

Cesarean rates also are examined for mothers who have "no indicated risk" (NIR) for cesarean delivery. This is a subgroup of United States births comprising the lowest-risk population identifiable from birth certificates: mothers who have full-term, singleton, vertex presentation births and none of the 16 medical risk factors (eg, diabetes, hypertension) or 15 labor and delivery complications (eg, fetal distress, prolonged labor) reported on birth certificates and no prior cesarean. Neonatal outcomes by method of delivery for low-risk women also are examined and available literature is reviewed.

Results

The percentage of United States births delivered by cesarean has increased by 50% in the past decade. In 2006, 31.1% of United States births were delivered by cesarean compared with 20.7% in 1996 (Fig. 1). The pace of the increase shows no signs of slowing, as increases are more rapid since 2000 [1,2]. The rapid increase in the cesarean rate reflects two concurrent trends: an increase in the primary cesarean rate and a steep decline in the VBAC rate (Fig. 2). The primary cesarean rate increased from 14.6% in 1996 to 20.6% in 2004. Sixty percent of the increase in the total cesarean rate from 1996 to 2004 was the result of increases in primary cesareans. At

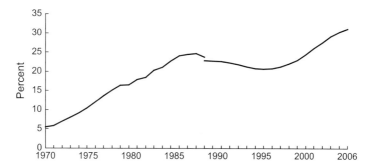

Fig. 1. Total cesarean delivery rate: United States, 1970–2006. (*Data from* Data for 1970–1988 are from the National Hospital Discharge Survey. Data for 1989–2006 are from the National Vital Statistics System, NCHS, Centers for Disease Control and Prevention [CDC]. Data for 2006 are preliminary.)

the same time, the VBAC rate decreased from 28.3% to 9.2%. A decrease in the VBAC rate implies a corresponding increase in the repeat cesarean rate, which reached almost 91% in 2004 [4]. Thus, the adage, "once a cesarean, always a cesarean," seems true for more than 90% of women in the United States.

National estimates of primary and repeat cesarean rates for 2005 and 2006 are not available because of a change in the wording and formatting of the method of delivery item on the 2003 revision of the United States Standard Certificate of Birth (used by 12 states in 2005) [2]. An examination of state-level data reveals, however, that primary and repeat cesarean rates continued to increase in 2005 [2]. The United States cesarean rate is high compared with that in many industrialized countries (Fig. 3); most developed countries, however, also have experienced increases over the past decade [5].

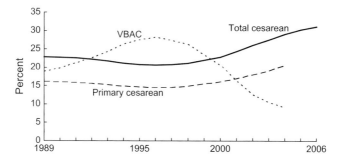

Fig. 2. Total cesarean delivery rate, United States, 1989–2006, and primary cesarean and VBAC Rates, 1989–2004. (*Data from* National Vital Statistics System, NCHS, CDC. Data for 2006 are preliminary.)

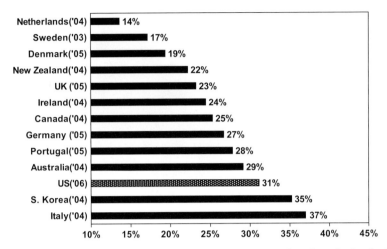

Fig. 3. Cesarean rates in industrialized countries, 2003–2006. (*Data from* Organization for Economic Cooperation and Development health data 2007; United States birth data for 2006 are preliminary.)

Variations by maternal age, race/ethnicity, gestational age, and state

Cesarean rates increase with increasing maternal age (Fig. 4). In 2006, nearly half (47.6%) of births among women ages 40 and over were delivered by cesarean compared with 22.2% of teen births. The higher rates for older mothers may be related to patient/practitioner concerns, increased rates of multiple births, and other biologic factors [6]. Still, for each maternal age group, cesarean rates increased sharply (by 45%–53%) from 1996 to 2006.

In 2006, cesarean rates were highest for non-Hispanic black women (33.1%), followed by non-Hispanic white (31.3%), Asian or Pacific Islander (30.6%), Hispanic (29.7%), and Native American women (27.4%) (Fig. 5).

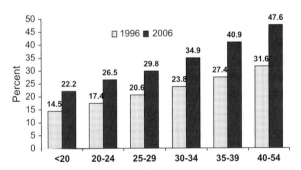

Fig. 4. Cesarean rates by age of mother: United States, 1996 and 2006. (*Data from* National Vital Statistics System, NCHS, CDC. Data for 2006 are preliminary.)

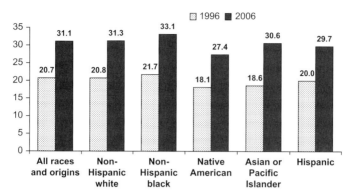

Fig. 5. Cesarean rates by race and Hispanic origin of mother: United States, 1996 and 2006. (*Data from* National Vital Statistics System, NCHS, CDC. Data for 2006 are preliminary.)

Cesarean rates increased rapidly from 1996 to 2006 for women of all race and ethnic groups. Increases were largest for Asian or Pacific Islander women (65%), followed by non-Hispanic black (53%), Native American (51%), non-Hispanic white (50%), and Hispanic women (49%).

Cesarean rates increased for births at all gestational ages between 1996 and 2005 (detailed data on cesarean delivery by gestational age for 2006 are not yet available) [2]. When only singleton births were examined (births in plural deliveries are more likely to be delivered by cesarean section), the trend was similar. The average annual increase in the cesarean rate at each gestational age category from 1997 to 1999 was 1% to 3%, compared with an average annual increase of 4% to 6% from 2000 to 2005. Between 1996 and 2005, cesarean rates rose by 33% to 50% for each gestational age category, including very preterm infants (<32 weeks of gestation) (Fig. 6). Cesarean rates were highest for very preterm infants. In 2005, nearly half

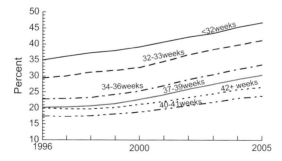

Fig. 6. Cesarean rates by gestational age, singleton births: United States, 1996–2005. (*Data from* National Vital Statistics System, NCHS, CDC.)

(46.8%) of very preterm singleton infants were delivered by cesarean. Approximately one third of singleton 34- to 36-week (late preterm) and 37- to 39-week infants were delivered by cesarean compared with approximately one quarter of singleton infants born at 40 weeks or greater.

In 2006, cesarean rates varied considerably by state, from a low of 21.5% in Utah to a high of 37.4% in New Jersey (Fig. 7) [1]. Although there is no clear-cut regional pattern, cesarean rates tended to be higher in the Southeastern states, selected Appalachian states, and some states on the Eastern Seaboard. Cesarean rates were lower in the Western Mountain and Upper Midwestern states. From 1996 to 2006, cesarean rates increased sharply in all states [1,2].

Questions and controversy generated by the increasing trends

The increasing trend in cesareans has generated controversy in the medical literature. Fundamental questions have been raised about the reasons for the increasing trend. Is the increase the result of changes in physician practice patterns regarding cesarean delivery, increases in maternal requests for cesarean section, or some combination of the two? Is the overall increase in the cesarean rate the result in part of increases in medically elective cesareans? Has there been a change in the medical risk profile of expectant mothers, such that more births are now at higher risk? And, finally, what are the benefits and harms of cesarean delivery for mothers and neonates?

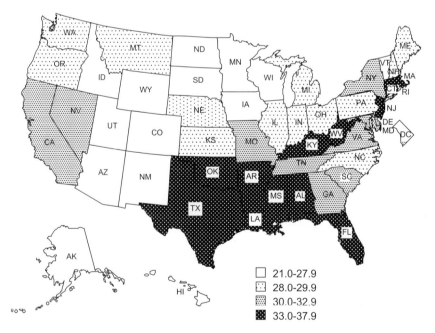

Fig. 7. Cesarean rates by state: United States, 2006. (*Data from* Preliminary data from the National Vital Statistics System, NCHS, CDC.)

Trends in the medical risk profile of mothers

Studies examining changes in the medical risk profile of mothers over time have found little evidence to suggest that the rising cesarean rates are due to such changes [7–10]. Declercq and colleagues [9] used birth certificate data to examine the medical risk profiles of women over time with regards to age, race/ethnicity, parity, gestational age, and birthweight and for a wide variety of medical risk factors and complications of labor or delivery. They found that changing primary cesarean rates were not related to general shifts in mothers' medical risk profiles. Rather, cesarean rates associated with virtually every demographic or medical risk factor reported on birth certificates shifted in the same pattern as with the overall cesarean rates. They concluded, "changes in obstetric practices were the major influence on the shifting pattern of primary cesarean rates" [9]. A related study used multivariate logistic regression analysis to examine changes in primary cesarean rates over time for NIR deliveries after controlling for parity; birthweight; and maternal ethnicity, age, and education and found that the odds of having a primary cesarean in 2001 were 50% higher than the odds in 1996 [7]. Similarly, Rhodes and colleagues [10] found that excess weight gain during pregnancy and macrosomia did not explain the increase in cesarean delivery as cesarean rates increased in all weight gain categories, and the incidence of macrosomia actually declined from 1990 to 2000.

Recent studies also have suggested that prepregnancy obesity (a measure currently not available from national birth certificate data) is related to higher primary cesarean rates [11,12]. (Information on maternal prepregnancy weight and weight gain is being collected on the 2003 revision of the birth certificate, but these data are not yet available in combination for all states.) Rates of obesity among United States women in all age groups increased, however, during the 1990s [13], whereas cesarean rates fell from 1991 to 1996 and then increased from 1996 to 2000. Conversely, obesity rates did not increase from 1999 to 2004 among United States women of reproductive age [14], whereas the cesarean rate continued to climb; thus, changes in obesity do not seem to be the primary driving force behind the increase in the cesarean rate.

Trends for women who have no indicated medical or obstetric risk
for cesarean

Studies estimating population-based trends in cesarean deliveries with no reported medical indications generally have used birth certificate data, hospital discharge data, or a combination of both. DeClercq and colleagues [7] used United States birth certificate data to identify a group of women who had NIR for cesarean delivery. These comprised full-term, singleton, vertex presentation births with no medical risk factors or complications of labor or delivery reported on the birth certificate and no prior cesarean. For this very low-risk group, the rate of primary cesareans has been rising since 1991 and especially rapidly since 1996 [7]. When data from this study were updated to

2003 [15], the overall primary cesarean rate for births to mothers who had NIR was 6.9%, nearly twice the 3.7% in 1996. The rate for first-time mothers was even higher, at 11.2% in 2003 (Fig. 8).

These results are comparable to those of other studies. Bailit and colleagues [16], using birth certificate data, estimated the primary cesarean delivery rate among women who had no medical or obstetric indication at approximately 7% in 2001. Two other recent studies used hospital discharge data to estimate the cesarean rate among women who had no reported medical or obstetric indication at 3% to 7% [17,18]. The methodology for the hospital discharge studies is similar to that for the birth certificate studies and involves identifying mothers who had low-risk births (full term or singletons) and no *International Classification of Disease* codes associated with labor or with complications of labor and delivery in their hospital discharge records [17,18]. A study that identified the subset of women who had NIR factors in birth certificate or hospital discharge data found a lower rate of medically elective cesareans (1.4%), based on 1998 to 2003 data [19]. Regardless of the exact level in a given year, all available studies document a recent rapid increase in cesarean delivery in low-risk women who had no medical indications for cesarean delivery.

Data on physician intention for method of delivery is not reported in birth certificate or hospital discharge data systems. Also, comparisons may be limited by possible under-reporting of medical risks and complications on birth certificates (see discussion later). Still, cesarean deliveries among low-risk women who have no medical indications represent the best approximation of a "medically elective" cesarean group possible from these large data sets.

Maternal opinions regarding cesarean delivery

The concept of maternal request cesarean has been defined variously in the medical literature. In some cases, it is defined simply as "primary elective

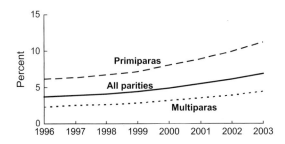

Fig. 8. Primary cesarean rates by parity for women who had NIR: United States, 1996–2003. NIR indicates women who had full-term vertex singleton births, birthweight less than 4000 g, and no reported medical risk factors or complications of labor or delivery. (*Data from* National Vital Statistics System, NCHS, CDC.)

cesarean delivery in the absence of a medical or obstetric indication" [20,21]. This definition, however, does not take into account the complex and nuanced interaction between an obstetric care provider and a patient in decision making. A recent review of studies on decision making surrounding cesarean delivery concluded, "the medical norms of health services . . . seem to drive nonmedically indicated cesarean delivery rates," and advocated for more detailed studies that examined patient-practitioner interactions within the context of care [22].

Despite widespread discussion in the medical literature about maternal request cesareans, few United States studies have asked pregnant women directly about their preferences for delivery method. *Listening to Mothers II* was a survey of 1573 mothers ages 18 to 45 who gave birth in a hospital to a singleton, still living infant in 2005. Results were weighted to reflect the national population [23]. In this study, for a mother to have a maternal request primary cesarean, she needed to meet two criteria: (1) have had the cesarean for no medical reason and (2) have made the decision for herself, before labor. Of the 252 mothers who had a primary cesarean in the survey, three indicated there was no medical indication for the cesarean and of these only one responded that she had made the decision to have a cesarean herself before beginning labor [23].

Results from the first *Listening to Mothers* survey, conducted in 2002, found little interest in a future elective primary cesarean, with only 6% of primiparous mothers interested in that option in the future [24]. A British national survey of mothers also found the phenomenon of maternal request cesareans to be rare [25]. Research from other countries with high cesarean rates, notably Brazil [26] and Chile [27], has found that rather than the cesarean rate being driven primarily by maternal demands, it is the interaction between mothers and their providers that leads to the decision to perform a cesarean without a clear medical indication. For example in Potter and colleagues' study in Brazil [26], more than 80% of primiparous mothers in the study anticipated a vaginal birth 1 month before their due date, yet almost half of these mothers (66% in private hospitals) ended up with a cesarean. Thus, although true maternal request cesareans doubtless occur, direct surveys of women seem to indicate that they are not numerous enough to account for the recent increase in the United States cesarean rate.

Neonatal and maternal outcomes by method of delivery

Several recent review articles have examined the risks and benefits of medically elective cesarean versus vaginal delivery for the mother and infant [28–33]. Several of these reviews were an outcome of the March 2006 National Institutes of Health (NIH) State-of-the-Science Conference: Cesarean Delivery on Maternal Request [31–33]. The NIH panel, after a systematic review of the literature, noted the lack of well-controlled studies for many outcomes of interest [34]; however, four findings were supported by at least a moderate level of evidence. Medically elective cesarean delivery (compared with the combination of planned vaginal and unplanned cesarean delivery) was associated with: (1) a decreased risk for maternal hemorrhage; (2) an increased risk for respiratory problems for infants; (3) greater complications in subsequent pregnancies, including uterine rupture and placental implantation problems, and (4) longer maternal hospital stays [34]. Several recent studies have corroborated these findings [19,35–39]. The NIH panel further noted that studies on neonatal and maternal mortality lacked statistical power and consistent methodologies to reliably assess the effect of the planned delivery route [34]. As maternal and neonatal mortality are rare events for low-risk women in developed countries, very large sample sizes often are needed to detect statistically significant differences.

Several studies published in 2006 and 2007, and thus not included in the NIH conference and other reviews, may have the potential to shed further light on these issues. MacDorman and colleagues [40] examined neonatal mortality using linked birth and infant death certificate data for 1998 to 2001 from 5.7 million births with NIR for cesarean delivery. They found that even in the most conservative model (excluding congenital anomalies and Apgar scores less than 4 and adjusting for sociodemographic and medical risk factors), the odds ratio for neonatal mortality for primary cesarean delivery was 2.02 (1.60–2.55) compared with vaginal delivery.

The NIH conference advocated using an "intention-to-treat" methodology to analyze outcome data by method of delivery [34]. Using this methodology, emergency cesareans performed after a woman is in labor are combined with vaginal births to create a "planned vaginal delivery" category, because the original intention was evidently a vaginal delivery. The "planned cesarean" category includes only those deliveries where a cesarean section was performed without labor. When the MacDorman and colleagues' [41] data were reanalyzed using this methodology, the neonatal mortality rate for the cesarean without labor category was 1.73 compared with 0.72 for the planned vaginal category. In the most conservative model (excluding congenital anomalies and Apgar scores less than 4 and adjusting for sociodemographic and medical risk factors), the odds ratio for neonatal mortality for cesarean without labor was 1.69 (1.35–2.11) compared with "planned vaginal" delivery [41].

Although using different methodologies and not all using the intention-to-treat framework, several other recent studies have examined maternal or neonatal mortality in relation to method of delivery. Villar and co-workers [42], in a Latin American study, found, for infants in cephalic presentations, an odds ratio of neonatal mortality for cesarean delivery of 1.9 (1.6–2.3) compared with vaginal deliveries. Betran and colleagues [43], in a global study of the relationship between method of delivery and maternal and neonatal mortality, found that for countries with overall cesarean rates below 15%, higher cesarean rates were correlated with lower maternal mortality. For countries with national cesarean rates above 15%, however, "higher cesarean rates are predominantly correlated with higher maternal mortality. A similar pattern is found for infant and neonatal mortality." These findings were corroborated by Villar and coworkers for Latin America [44]. Other recent studies found increased risks for maternal mortality for low-risk women delivered by cesarean [45,46], whereas an additional study found substantial serious maternal morbidity associated with cesarean section but no significant difference in maternal mortality [39].

Discussion

Cesarean rates in the United States fell between 1991 and 1996 and then began to rise rapidly. In 2006, nearly one third (31.1%) of United States births were cesarean deliveries. Over the past decade, cesarean rates increased sharply for women of all ages, all race/ethnic groups, all periods of gestation and in all states. Cesarean rates were highest for women ages 35 and over, for non-Hispanic black women, and for preterm births. Sixty percent of the increase in the cesarean rate from 1996 to 2004 was the result of increases in the primary cesarean rate. Based on the trend in the repeat cesarean rate, a first cesarean delivery now virtually guarantees that subsequent deliveries will be cesarean deliveries. Repeat cesarean deliveries are associated with significantly higher maternal and neonatal morbidity and mortality compared with cesarean or vaginal deliveries for women who do not have a prior cesarean [34,36–38,47–48]. For example, in one study, the odds ratios of having a life-threatening placenta accreta were 2.4 (1.3–4.3) for a third cesarean and 9.0 (4.8–16.7) for a fourth cesarean compared with a primary cesarean [47,48].

Primary cesarean rates also have increased rapidly for women who have NIR for cesarean delivery, which is the closest approximation to a medically elective cesarean group available from birth certificates. Although comparisons are limited by differences in methodology between various studies, there seems to be more evidence now than at the time of the NIH conference for an increased risk for maternal and neonatal mortality and morbidity for medically elective cesareans compared with vaginal births. In addition, the increase in the primary cesarean rate seems primarily the result of changes in obstetric practice and not to changes in the medical risk profile of births or increases in maternal request.

Strengths of the birth certificate data to track trends in cesarean delivery include the comprehensive population-based nature of these data, which include all births in the United States for a given year. Most demographic items and some medical items (including maternal age and parity and method of delivery) are considered well reported [49,50]. There are limitations with regard to a measure of no indicated medical or obstetric risk. There has been documentation of under-reporting of medical risk factors and complications of labor and delivery on birth certificates [49–51]. Reporting a risk factor or complication associated with a resulting cesarean, however, would be expected to be encouraged. Also, there is no reason to suspect that the reporting of these variables has changed systematically over the past decade, potentially biasing trend analysis [9]. Unfortunately, future research using birth certificate data to identify NIR women will be further limited by differences in the specific risk factor data collected between the 1989 and 2003 revisions of the United States Standard Certificate of Birth. Because of the staggered implementation of the 2003 revision among states, both revisions are in use in different states, making it difficult to construct national estimates for the NIR group [1,2,52].

Discussions of the reasons for the growth in primary cesareans have centered on changing attitudes concerning cesareans among physicians and mothers [53–56]. Leitch and Walker [56] related the rise in the cesarean rate to a change in medical practice and concluded that although indications for cesarean did not change much over time, "there has been a lowering in the overall threshold concerning the decision to carry out a caesarean section." This, combined with the increase in medically elective cesareans, probably accounts for much of the increase in the cesarean rate over the past decade. A more detailed examination is needed of mother, insurer, hospital, and provider attitudes toward medically elective cesareans and of the nature of the interaction between mothers and their obstetric care providers in decision making about the method of delivery. Research on the economic implications of the rising cesarean rate for hospitals, providers, insurers, and parents also is essential.

There are markedly different practice recommendations regarding cesarean delivery from American and international obstetric groups. In discussing the ethics of medically elective cesareans, the American College of Obstetricians and Gynecologists states [54],

> In the absence of significant data on the risks and benefits of cesarean delivery…if the physician believes that cesarean delivery promotes the overall health and welfare of the woman and her fetus more than vaginal birth, he or she is ethically justified in performing a cesarean delivery.

In contrast, the International Federation of Gynecology and Obstetrics states [57],

> At present, because hard evidence of net benefit does not exist, performing cesarean section for non-medical reasons is not ethically justified.

In 2004, Queenan [58] noted that the underlying "question is not the ethics of patient choice, but lack of scientific proof of risks and benefits." It is hoped that with an increasing body of research on the harms and benefits of medically elective cesarean versus vaginal delivery, decision making regarding medically elective cesarean versus vaginal delivery will be increasingly evidence based.

References

[1] Hamilton BE, Martin JA, Ventura SJ. Births: preliminary data for 2006. National vital statistics reports, vol. 56 no 7. Hyattsville (MD): National Center for Health Statistics; 2007.

[2] Martin JA, Hamilton BE, Sutton PD, et al. Births: final data for 2005. National vital statistics reports, vol. 56 no 6. Hyattsville (MD): National Center for Health Statistics; 2007.

[3] DeFrances CJ, Hall MJ. 2005 National Hospital Discharge Survey. Advance data from vital and health statistics no 385. Hyattsville (MD): National Center for Health Statistics; 2007.

[4] Martin JA, Hamilton BE, Sutton PD, et al. Births: final data for 2004. National vital statistics reports, vol. 55 no 1. Hyattsville (MD): National Center for Health Statistics; 2006.

[5] Organization for Economic Cooperation and Development. OECD health data 2007: statistics and indicators for 30 countries 2007. Available at: http://www.oecd.org/document/30/0,2340,en_2649_34631_12968734_1_1_1_1,00.html. Accessed December 10, 2007.

[6] Ecker JL, Chen KT, Cohen AP, et al. Increased risk of cesarean delivery with advancing maternal age: indications and associated factors in nulliparous women. Am J Obstet Gynecol 2001;185:883–7.

[7] Declercq E, Menacker F, MacDorman MF. Rise in "no indicated risk" primary cesareans in the United States. 1991–2001. BMJ 2005;330:71–2.

[8] Reddy UM, Spong DY. Introduction. Semin Perinatol 2006;30:233–4.

[9] Declercq E, Menacker F, MacDorman MF. Maternal risk profiles and the primary cesarean rate in the United States, 1991–2002. Am J Public Health 2006;96:867–72.

[10] Rhodes JC, Schoendorf KC, Parker JD. Contribution of excess weight gain during pregnancy and macrosomia to the cesarean delivery rate, 1990–2000. Pediatrics 2003;111:1181–6.

[11] Lu GC, Rouse DJ, DuBard M, et al. The effect of the increasing prevalence of maternal obesity on perinatal morbidity. Am J Obstet Gynecol 2001;185:845–9.

[12] Kaiser PS, Kirby RS. Obesity as a risk factor for cesarean in a low risk population. Obstet Gynecol 2001;97:39–43.

[13] Flegal KM, Carroll MD, Ogden CL, et al. Prevalence and trends in obesity among US adults, 1999–2000. JAMA 2002;288:1723–7.

[14] Ogden CL, Carroll MD, Curtin LF, et al. Prevalence of overweight and obesity in the United States, 1999–2004. JAMA 2006;295:1549–55.

[15] Menacker F, Declercq E, MacDorman MF. Cesarean delivery: background, trends and epidemiology. Semin Perinatol 2006;30:235–41.

[16] Bailit JL, Love TE, Mercer B. Rising cesarean rates: are patients sicker? Am J Obstet Gynecol 2004;191:800–1.

[17] Gregory KD, Korst LM, Gornbein JA, et al. Using administrative data to identify indications for elective cesarean delivery. Health Serv Res 2002;37:1387–401.

[18] Healthgrades. Healthgrades third annual report on "patient-choice" Cesarean section rates in the United States. Available at: http://www.healthgrades.com. Accessed September, 2005.

[19] Declercq E, Barger M, Cabral HJ, et al. Maternal outcomes associated with planned primary cesarean births compared with planned vaginal births. Obstet Gynecol 2007;109:669–77.

[20] Wax JR, Cartin A, Pinette MG, et al. Patient choice cesarean: an evidence-based review. Obstet Gynecol Surv 2004;59:601–16.

[21] Gossman GL, Joesch JM, Tanfer K. Trends in maternal request cesarean delivery from 1991 to 2004. Obstet Gynecol 2006;108:1506–16.

[22] Gamble J, Creedy DK, McCourt C, et al. A critique of the literature on women's request for cesarean section. Birth 2007;34:331–40.

[23] Declercq ER, Sakala C, Corry MP, et al. Listening to mothers II—report of the second national U.S. survey of women's childbearing experiences, October 2006. New York: Childbirth Connection; Available at: http://www.childbirthconnection.org/article.asp?ck=10401. Accessed December 10, 2007.

[24] Declercq ER, Sakala C, et al. Listening to mothers: report of the First National U.S. Survey of women's childbearing experiences, October 2002. New York. Maternity Center Association; Available at: http://www.childbirthconnection.org/pdfs/LtMreport.pdf. Accessed December 10, 2007.

[25] Redshaw M, Rowe R, Hockley C, et al. Recorded delivery: a national survey of women's experience with maternity care, 2006. Oxford: National Perinatal Epidemiology Unit; 2007.

[26] Potter JE, Berquó E, Perpétuo IHO, et al. Unwanted caesarean sections among public and private patients in Brazil: prospective study. BMJ 2001;323:1155–8.

[27] Murray SF. Relation between private health insurance and high rates of caesarean section in Chile: qualitative and quantitative study. BMJ 2000;321:1501–5.

[28] Visco AG, Viswanathan M, Lohr K, et al. Cesarean delivery on maternal request—maternal and neonatal outcomes. Obstet Gynecol 2006;108:1517–29.

[29] Doherty EG, Eichenwald EC. Cesarean delivery: emphasis on the neonate. Clin Obstet Gynecol 2004;47:332–41.

[30] Lavender T, Hofmeyr GJ, Neilson JP, et al. Caesarean section for non-medical reasons at term [review]. Cochrane Database Syst Rev 2006;3:CD004660.

[31] Signore D, Hemachandra A, Klebanoff M. Neonatal mortality and morbidity after elective cesarean delivery versus routine expectant management: a decision analysis. Semin Perinatol 2006;30:288–95.

[32] Wax JR. Maternal request cesarean versus planned spontaneous vaginal delivery: maternal morbidity and short term outcomes. Semin Perinatol 2006;30:247–52.

[33] Vadnais M, Sachs B. Maternal mortality with cesarean delivery: a literature review. Semin Perinatol 2006;30:242–6.

[34] NIH State-of-the-Science Conference statement on cesarean delivery on maternal request. NIH Consens State Sci statements. 2006;23(1):1–29. Available at: http://consensus.nih.gov/2006/2006CesareanSOS027main.htm. Accessed April 10, 2008.

[35] Kolas T, Saugstad OD, Daltveit AK, et al. Planned cesarean versus planned vaginal delivery at term: comparison of newborn infant outcomes. Am J Obstet Gynecol 2006;195:1538–43.

[36] Yang Q, Wen SW, Oppenheimer L, et al. Association of caesarean delivery for first birth with placenta praevia and placental abruption in second pregnancy. BJOG 2007;114:609–13.

[37] Kennare R, Tucker G, Heard A, et al. Risks of adverse outcomes in the next birth after a first cesarean delivery. Obstet Gynecol 2007;109:270–6.

[38] Spong DY, Landon MB, Gilbert S, et al. Risk of uterine repution and adverse perinatal outcome at term after cesarean delivery. Obstet Gynecol 2007;110:801–7.

[39] Liu S, Liston RM, Joseph KS, et al. Maternal mortality and severe morbidity associated with low-risk planned cesarean delivery versus planned vaginal delivery at term. CMAJ 2007;176:455–60.

[40] MacDorman MF, Declercq E, Menacker F, et al. Infant and neonatal mortality for primary cesarean and vaginal births to women with "no indicated risk," United States, 1998–2001 birth cohorts. Birth 2006;33:175–82.

[41] MacDorman MF, Declercq E, Menacker F , et al. Neonatal mortality for primary cesarean and vaginal births to low-risk women: application of an "intention-to-treat" model. Birth 2008;35(1):3–8.

[42] Villar J, Carroli G, Zavaleta N, et al. Maternal and neonatal individual risks and benefits associated with caesarean delivery: multicenter prospective study. BMJ 2007;1025–35 [published online first].

[43] Betran AP, Merialdi M, Lauer JA, et al. Rates of caesarean section: analysis of global, regional and national estimates. Paediatr Perinat Epidemiol 2007;21:98–113.

[44] Villar J, VAlladares E, Wojdyla D, et al. Caesarean delivery rates and pregnancy outcomes: the 2005 WHO global survey on maternal and perinatal health in Latin America. Lancet 2006;367:1819–29.

[45] Deneux-Tharaux C, Carmona E, Bouvier-Colle MH, et al. Postpartum maternal mortality and cesarean delivery. Obstet Gynecol 2006;108:541–8.

[46] Schutte JM, Steegers EAP, Santema JG, et al. Maternal deaths after elective cesarean section for breech presentation in the Netherlands. Acta Obstet Gynecol Scand 2007;86:240–3.

[47] Silver RM, Landon MB, Rouse DJ, et al. Maternal morbidity associated with multiple repeat cesarean deliveries. Obstet Gynecol 2006;107:1226–32.

[48] American College of Obstetricians and Gynecologists, Committee on Obstetric Practice. Cesarean delivery on maternal request. ACOG Committee Opinion number 394, December 2007. Obstet Gynecol 2007;110:1501–4.

[49] Roohan PJ, Josberger RE, Acar J, et al. Validation of birth certificate data in New York State. J Community Health 2003;28:335–46.

[50] DiGiuseppe DL, Aron DC, Ranbom L, et al. Reliability of birth certificate data: a multi-hospital comparison to medical records information. Matern Child Health J 2002;6:169–79.

[51] Lydon-Rochelle MT, Holt VL, Cardenas V, et al. The reporting of pre-existing maternal medical conditions and complications of pregnancy on birth certificates and in hospital discharge data. Am J Obstet Gynecol 2005;193:125–34.

[52] Hamilton BE, Minino AM, Martin JA, et al. Annual summary of vital statistics: 2005-Pediatrics 2007;119:345–60.

[53] Minkoff H, Powderly KR, Chervenak F, et al. Ethical dimensions of elective primary cesarean delivery. Obstet Gynecol 2004;103:387–92.

[54] American College of Obstetricians and Gynecologists. Surgery and patient choice. In: Ethics in obstetrics and gynecology. 2nd edition. Washington, DC: The American College of Obstetricians and Gynecologists; 2004. p. 21.

[55] Hale RW, Harer WB. Elective prophylactic cesarean delivery [editorial]. ACOG Clin Rev 2005;10(2):1–15.

[56] Leitch CR, Walker JJ. The rise in caesarean section rate: the same indications but a lower threshold. Br J Obstet Gynaecol 1998;105:621–6.

[57] Issues in Obstetrics and Gynecology by The FIGO Committee for the Ethical Aspects Of Human Reproduction And Women's Health. 41-2, (1998), 2003. Available at: http://www.figo.org/docs/Ethics%20Guidelines.pdf. Accessed December 10, 2007.

[58] Queenan JT. Elective cesarean delivery. Obstet Gynecol 2004;103:1135–6.

ELSEVIER
SAUNDERS

CLINICS IN
PERINATOLOGY

Clin Perinatol 35 (2008) 309–323

The Relationship Between Cesarean Delivery and Gestational Age Among US Singleton Births

Vani R. Bettegowda, MHS[a],*, Todd Dias, MS[a],
Michael J. Davidoff, MPH[a], Karla Damus, RN, PhD[b],
William M. Callaghan, MD, MPH[c],
Joann R. Petrini, PhD, MPH[a,b]

[a]*Perinatal Data Center, National Office, March of Dimes Foundation,
1275 Mamaroneck Avenue, White Plains, NY 10605, USA*
[b]*Department of Obstetrics, Gynecology, and Women's Health, Albert Einstein
College of Medicine, 1300 Morris Park Avenue, Bronx, NY 10461, USA*
[c]*Division of Reproductive Health, National Center for Chronic Disease Prevention
and Health Promotion, Centers for Disease Control and Prevention,
4770 Buford Highway, MS K-23, Atlanta, GA 30341, USA*

The recent significant left shift of the gestational age distribution for singleton births in the United States [1] has catalyzed concerns about the implications for maternal and infant health. Increased obstetric interventions to better manage high-risk pregnancies, including those occurring post-term, are part of this trend, but questions about iatrogenic preterm delivery are more challenging to answer because of limitations of extant data sources. Given the growing national toll of preterm birth (less than 37 completed weeks gestation) [2], it is imperative to determine the contribution of modifiable factors so that, if feasible, some early births can be prevented. This requires a better understanding of the convergence of changes in: the distribution of gestational age at birth; rates of adverse perinatal outcomes, such as preterm birth and perinatal mortality; and clinical management practices, including obstetric interventions for which reliable data are available, such as method of delivery.

The findings and conclusions in this report are those of the authors and do not necessarily represent the views of the respective agencies.

* Corresponding author.

E-mail address: vbettegowda@marchofdimes.com (V.R. Bettegowda).

Although most singleton births in the United States continue to be delivered vaginally, 30.3% of births in 2005 (1.2 million) [3] were delivered by primary or repeat cesarean section, making cesarean section the most common major surgical procedure for women in the United States [4]. Given that both primary and repeat cesarean deliveries have increased in recent years, the total cesarean section rate provides an acceptable measure for tracking this obstetric intervention over time. The leading obstetric problem in the nation, preterm birth, has also increased. Since 1981, the preterm birth rate has increased more than 30% reaching an all time high of 12.7% in 2005, which means that approximately 1 in 8 births was preterm [3]. Although the increasing rate of multiple births has contributed to the increase in preterm births, 83% of babies born early in 2004 were singletons [5].

The nation's increase in preterm births is of great clinical and public health concern. Preterm births, particularly at the earliest gestational ages, are the leading contributor to neonatal morbidity and mortality in the United States, and national cost estimates for the first several years of life are estimated to exceed $26 billion annually [2,6,7]. Prevention of "preventable" preterm births is therefore of high priority, and potential amenable contributors require study and interpretation. Previous analyses have revealed that more recent increases in the US preterm birth rate were almost exclusively driven by increases in late preterm births (34–36 weeks) [1] and were associated with a parallel increase in medically indicated preterm birth [8,9]. Because these late preterm births have significant morbidity, the American College of Obstetricians and Gynecologists (ACOG) cautions against elective induction and cesarean delivery before 39 weeks without evidence of fetal maturity [10,11]. However, increases in obstetric interventions appear to be shifting gestational ages earlier [1,12]. Analyzing the relationship among these contemporaneous trends in perinatal outcomes and method of delivery will provide insights about the increasing preterm birth rate and potential strategies for its reduction. This article explores the relationship of cesarean delivery and the changing distribution of gestational age among singleton live births in the United States, focusing on the increasing rates of cesarean delivery and preterm births between 1996 and 2004.

Trends in cesarean delivery

The total cesarean section rate rose sharply in the 1970s and 1980s, accounting for only 5% of live births in 1970 and nearly 25% of all deliveries in 1988 [13,14]. Medically indicated cesarean delivery can avert complications and adverse outcomes for the pregnant woman and fetus. However, compared with vaginal delivery cesarean section is associated with increased maternal morbidity, hospital readmission, longer hospital stays, and higher health care costs [15–23]. There can also be potential risks for infants delivered by cesarean section, such as laceration, neonatal respiratory problems, and iatrogenic prematurity [9,24–26]. Furthermore, maternal risks in subsequent pregnancies after a cesarean section delivery include uterine rupture, placenta previa, placenta accreta, and hysterectomy [17,27,28]. Weighing the benefits, potential risks, and increasing rates, national organizations, including the National Institutes of Health and ACOG, encouraged measures to decrease cesarean delivery unless medically necessary and to increase vaginal birth after cesarean (VBAC) [29,30]. Between 1989 and 1995, there was a decline in the cesarean section rate [3,29]. However, during this period many factors were changing. There were more high-risk pregnancies and reports of complications associated with VBAC [3,31]. This led to increasing concerns about safety [29,32,33] and, eventually, to a sharp reduction in VBAC rates paralleled by an increase in the cesarean section rate [29].

Between 1996 and 2005, the cesarean section rate increased 46%, from 20.7% to 30.3% of live births [3]. This largely reflects a sharp increase in primary cesarean section rates, which may further increase subsequent cesarean delivery rates considering that women who have a primary cesarean section are increasingly likely to be delivered by repeat cesarean section [3,34]. Cesarean section rates also vary by maternal race/ethnicity, with the highest cesarean section rates for women who were non-Hispanic black (32.6%), followed by non-Hispanic white (30.4%) and Hispanic (29.0%) women. Between 1996 and 2005, these rates have increased substantially for all maternal racial/ethnic groups, with an increase of 50% for non-Hispanic black women, 46% for non-Hispanic white women, and 45% for Hispanic women [3]. The increasing rates of cesarean delivery provide a picture of changing maternal risks and obstetric practice patterns in the United States.

Trends in preterm birth

The total preterm birth rate has increased more than 30% over the past two decades, from 9.4% of live births in 1981 to 12.7% in 2005. Between 1993 and 1996, the preterm birth rate was unchanged at 11%. In 1997, as the cesarean section rates began to increase again, the preterm birth rate increased to 11.4% and rose steadily, except for a small decrease from 11.8% to 11.6% between 1999 and 2000. Preterm birth rates differed by maternal race/ethnicity, and in 2005, non-Hispanic black infants were nearly twice as likely to be born preterm as non-Hispanic white and Hispanic infants (18.4% versus 11.7% and 12.1%, respectively). While preterm birth rates for non-Hispanic white infants have increased steadily in the past decade, preterm birth rates for non-Hispanic black infants began to increase in 2001 after a period of decline in the 1990s [3].

Between 1981 and 2005, the very preterm (less than 32 completed weeks gestation) birth rate remained relatively stable at approximately 2%, whereas the late preterm birth rate increased more than 44% (from 6.3% to 9.1%) [3,35]. Currently, late preterm infants comprise more than 70% of all preterm births in the United States and are the fastest growing subgroup of preterm births [1,3]. The rising rate of late preterm birth has been shown to be associated, in part, with increasing obstetric intervention [9]. Further, evidence supporting adverse outcomes among late preterm births is also growing.

Growing concerns about late preterm birth

Recent research has focused on late preterm births and revealed higher incidences of neonatal complications when compared with term births. Late preterm infants have elevated risks for respiratory distress syndrome, transient tachypnea of the newborn, hypoglycemia, temperature instability, jaundice, and feeding difficulties [36–39]. Recently, McIntire and Leveno [40] reported that neonatal morbidity rates decreased significantly with increasing gestational age between 34 and 39 weeks. Morbidities included ventilator-treated respiratory distress, transient tachypnea, grade 1 or 2 intraventricular hemorrhage, sepsis workups, culture-proved sepsis, phototherapy, and intubation in the delivery room. Late preterm infants also required more resources with longer lengths of hospital stay and higher hospital costs associated with admission to neonatal intensive care units (NICUs) and were more likely to be rehospitalized after discharge [40–43].

The risk of infant mortality is also higher for late preterm infants compared with term infants. In 2004, the infant mortality rate among late preterm infants was three times higher than among term infants (7.3 versus 2.4 infant deaths per 1,000 live births) [44,45]. This disparity is greater in the neonatal period and in the first week of life [40,45]. When causes of death reported in linked birth/infant death records were assessed, higher neonatal mortality rates were attributable to pregnancy complications and birth defects that required early delivery rather than attributed to the early delivery itself. However, even when birth defects were excluded as a cause of death, the infant mortality rates continued to be threefold higher for late preterm compared with term infants [45].

Changing patterns of singleton gestational age and delivery method

Analyses of the 1996 and 2004 US natality files were conducted to shed more light on the trends in cesarean section and the timing of delivery. All analyses were limited to singleton live births. Records were excluded if method of delivery, gestational age, or birth weight was unknown; if gestational age was less than 23 weeks or greater than 44 weeks; or if birth weight was less than 500 g.

Method of delivery was classified as vaginal or cesarean section. Vaginal deliveries included VBAC deliveries, and cesarean deliveries included primary and repeat sections. Despite the known relationship between some cases of cesarean delivery and labor induction, the underreported rates of induction precluded any reliable detailed analyses and are not presented [46,47].

Gestational age reported in the natality file as completed weeks of gestation was based on the period between the first day of the mother's last normal menstrual period and the infant's date of birth. Gestational age was stratified a priori into seven groups by completed gestational week: <32, 32 and 33, 34 to 36, 37 and 38, 39, 40 and 41, and 42 to 44 weeks. Gestational age group–specific cesarean section rates were calculated for non-Hispanic white, non-Hispanic black, and Hispanic maternal race/ethnicity groups.

Preterm birth and method of delivery

Preterm birth rates among singletons (total, vaginal, and cesarean) for 1996 and 2004 are presented in Table 1. While the singleton preterm birth rates have increased for both vaginal and cesarean deliveries, the change over time in the respective rates was the result of whether and how much both the numerators (number of singleton preterm births by method of delivery) as well as the denominators (number of singleton births by method of delivery) changed. These changes influenced all rates. During the study period, the numerator rose much more than the denominator, thereby increasing the overall singleton preterm birth rate (see *Total* column). When considered with the results in the *Vaginal* and *Cesarean* columns, it is reasonable to conclude that the singleton preterm birth rate increased among vaginal and cesarean deliveries. However, close inspection of the respective numerators and denominators suggests that vaginal preterm birth rates increased for different reasons than the cesarean preterm birth rates.

Among singleton vaginal deliveries, the preterm birth rate increased from 9.0% of live births in 1996 to 9.6% in 2004. However, the increase in the preterm birth rate among vaginal singletons was driven by the large *decrease* of 141,732 vaginal births rather than the relatively small increase of 4,652 preterm vaginal births. In contrast, the increase in the preterm birth rate for singleton cesarean deliveries from 12.7% in 1996 to 13.6% in 2004 was primarily driven by the increase in preterm births, as there were increases in the numerator and denominator. Furthermore, the number of preterm births increased by 59,057, and 54,405 of those were delivered by cesarean section, reflecting a cesarean-to-vaginal delivery ratio of more than 11 to 1.

Table 1
Preterm birth rates among singleton vaginal and cesarean section births, 1996 and 2004

		Total			Vaginal			Cesarean section	
	1996	2004	Absolute difference	1996	2004	Absolute difference	1996	2004	Absolute difference
Preterm (numerator)	354,997	414,054	59,057	263,520	268,172	4,652	91,477	145,882	54,405
Total births (denominator)	3,666,960	3,873,554	206,594	2,944,204	2,802,472	−141,732	722,756	1,071,082	348,326
Preterm birth rate	9.7%	10.7%	1.0%	9.0%	9.6%	0.6%	12.7%	13.6%	0.9%

To further understand the concurrently changing patterns of delivery method and gestational age in the United States, singleton births were stratified into four mutually exclusive groups: vaginal preterm, cesarean preterm, vaginal not preterm, and cesarean not preterm (Fig. 1). Between 1996 and 2004, the proportion of singleton preterm births that were delivered vaginally decreased from 7.2% to 6.9% (–0.3%) while the proportion of preterm births that were delivered by cesarean increased from 2.5% to 3.8% (+1.3%), resulting in an absolute increase of 1% in the overall singleton preterm birth rate from 9.7% to 10.7%.

To provide greater detail of the categorical data in Fig. 1, the continuous gestational week distribution by delivery method was graphed in Fig. 2. At each week, the denominator is all singleton births, such that at any given week, the vaginal and cesarean percentages add up to the total proportion of all singleton births at that gestational week. Among cesarean section births, there was a left shift in the shoulder of the distribution curve toward earlier gestational weeks. Notably, for late preterm births, there was no increase in the proportion of births delivered vaginally, but a marked increase in the proportion of births delivered by cesarean section. Overall, these results show that the increase in the preterm birth rate, especially for late preterm births, occurred primarily among cesarean section deliveries.

Cesarean section rates by gestational age and maternal race/ethnicity

Additional analyses were done to assess changes in the singleton cesarean section rates by gestational age and maternal race/ethnicity. Between 1996 and 2004, singleton cesarean section rates increased at each gestational

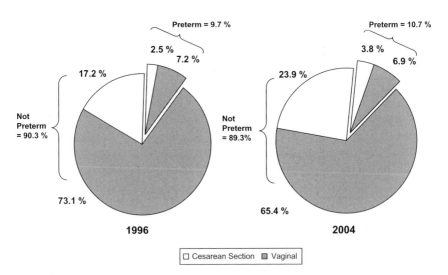

Fig. 1. Distribution of singleton live births by preterm and not preterm and method of delivery, 1996 and 2004.

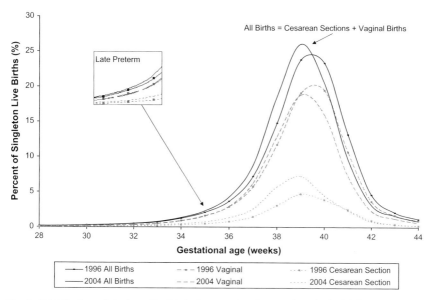

Fig. 2. Distribution of singleton live births by gestational age and method of delivery, 1996 and 2004.

week (Fig. 3). Cesarean section rates have also increased for each gestational age group for all maternal race/ethnicity groups (Table 2). Each group showed a similar pattern with larger percentage increases in the middle gestational age groups. Non-Hispanic black women experienced the largest percentage increases, with rates in 2004 reaching levels experienced by non-Hispanic white women. Fig. 4 shows that non-Hispanic black women had much larger increases in the preterm gestational age groups. These increases have negated the historical differences in cesarean section rates between non-Hispanic black and non-Hispanic white women. Although the reasons for this observation are not clear, recent evidence of differences in gestational age misclassification between non-Hispanic blacks and non-Hispanic whites may be partly responsible [48]. Among preterm births, the largest percentage increase in cesarean section rates occurred in the late preterm group, which is the largest and fastest growing segment of preterm births.

Indications for cesarean deliveries associated with preterm birth

The frequency of early cesarean delivery is increasing for medical/obstetric indications and when warranted for logistic reasons, such as risk of rapid labor or distance from a hospital [8–10]. For many of these cases, this reflects optimal management, such as when attempting to prevent or manage fetal distress, maternal bleeding, infections, or severe preeclampsia. Given the state of available information, several important questions should

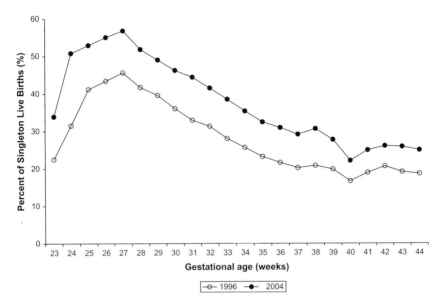

Fig. 3. Gestational age–specific cesarean section rates among singleton live births, 1996 and 2004. (*Adapted from* Davidoff MJ, Dias T, Damus K, et al. Changes in the gestational age distribution among US singleton births: impact on rates of late preterm birth, 1992 to 2002. Semin Perinatol 2006;30:12; with permission.)

be posed. First, can the increased proportion of medically complicated pregnancies explain most of the increases in cesarean section rates? Alternatively, are interventions (including cesarean sections) occurring earlier in gestation and substantially contributing to increases in preterm birth rates? Finally, if cesarean sections without medical or obstetric indications are being performed before term, can they be prevented? These questions will be addressed in the following sections.

Medical/obstetric indications for cesarean delivery

Changes in demographics and medical risks have been evaluated as proposed contributors to the increase in the primary cesarean section rate [49,50]. Declercq and colleagues [49] examined demographic and medical risk factors between 1991 and 2002 and revealed no association between changes in the maternal risk profile and shifts in the primary cesarean section rates. However, this study was based on birth certificate data and the underreporting of pregnancy complications is well documented [49,51–53]. Obesity among women of childbearing age has been reported to be associated with cesarean delivery [54,55] and suggested to relate to increasing cesarean section rates [56,57]. However, obesity rates have climbed steadily in the past two decades, but the overall cesarean section pattern has been one of decline and increase beginning in the mid-1990s [49,58].

Table 2
Change in singleton cesarean section rates by gestational age groups and maternal race/ethnicity, 1996 and 2004

Gestational age (weeks)	1996	2004	Percent change
All singleton live births			
<32	37.4	48.6	30
32 and 33	29.4	39.7	35
34 to 36	22.8	32.1	41
37 and 38	20.6	30.1	46
39	19.8	27.7	40
40 and 41	17.5	23.0	31
42 to 44	19.9	25.8	30
Non-Hispanic white			
<32	41.4	50.6	22
32 and 33	33.1	42.9	30
34 to 36	24.3	33.2	37
37 and 38	21.5	30.8	43
39	20.2	27.9	38
40 and 41	16.8	22.1	32
42 to 44	19.6	25.4	30
Non-Hispanic black			
<32	33.2	47.4	43
32 and 33	25.1	37.5	49
34 to 36	20.7	31.3	51
37 and 38	19.4	29.4	52
39	20.0	29.0	45
40 and 41	20.7	27.2	31
42 to 44	21.8	28.7	32
Hispanic			
<32	35.8	46.6	30
32 and 33	27.5	36.4	32
34 to 36	21.6	30.9	43
37 and 38	20.0	29.6	48
39	18.9	26.8	42
40 and 41	17.6	22.8	30
42 to 44	19.9	25.3	27

Davidoff and colleagues [1] looked at the changing distribution of singleton live births and found increasing rates of cesarean section and induction of labor contributing to the shift to earlier gestational ages that was not explained by changes in demographic characteristics, such as maternal race/ethnicity and maternal age. Between 1992 and 2002, the proportion of spontaneous deliveries and deliveries with premature rupture of membranes (PROM) declined, while there was an increase in births delivered by medical intervention from 29% in 1992 to 41% in 2002. Similarly, a study by Ananth and colleagues [8] examined trends in preterm birth by delivery category between 1989 and 2000 and found that spontaneous preterm birth and preterm birth resulting from PROM declined, whereas medically indicated preterm birth increased from 2.6% to 3.8%.

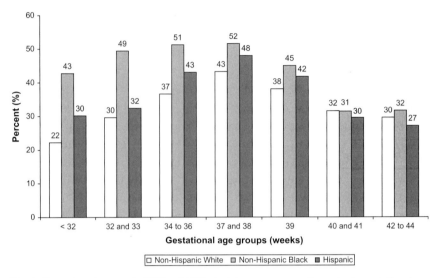

Fig. 4. Percentage increase in 1996 and 2004 singleton cesarean section rates by gestational age groups and maternal race/ethnicity.

Ananth and colleagues [8] also reported that more than 30% of singleton preterm births were medically indicated. In a separate study, maternal and fetal conditions requiring medical interventions that resulted in iatrogenic preterm birth were evaluated [59]. Conditions associated with ischemic placental disease, such as preeclampsia, fetal distress, small for gestational age, and placental abruption, were implicated in more than half of medically indicated preterm births [59]. Although this study was based on birth certificate data, other clinical studies have supported the observation that one of these four conditions was present in the majority of preterm births that required medical intervention [60,61]. With respect to preeclampsia, expectant management should be considered for women who have mild preeclampsia [62]. For those with severe preeclampsia, management is best accomplished in a tertiary facility or with consultation of a high-risk obstetrician-gynecologist with delivery as needed [62]. An increased incidence of preterm birth has been reported among women with gestational hypertension or preeclampsia [63,64]. Addressing preeclampsia and late preterm birth, Fuchs and Wapner [65] recommend delivery at 37 weeks for mild preeclampsia and as early as 34 weeks for severe preeclampsia. Pregnancy complications increase the opportunity for iatrogenic preterm birth, but the extent of their contribution to increasing preterm birth rates requires further investigation.

Non-medical/obstestric indications for cesarean delivery

There are emerging ethical and clinical concerns that some early deliveries may occur for non-medically indicated reasons, such as convenience and patient preference. It is estimated that 2.5% of all US births are delivered by cesarean section on maternal request [21]. In 2005, this translated to approximately 103,000 live births [3]. Birth certificate data do not include information to distinguish between medically indicated and patient choice cesarean section; therefore, the contribution of elective cesarean delivery to the rising total cesarean section rate is unknown [3,21]. McCourt and colleagues [66] reported that there is little evidence of women requesting cesarean sections. However, several studies reviewed suggest that provider preferences and perceptions of women's views may play a role in delivery decision making [66].

Studies on neonatal outcomes and cesarean section on maternal request are lacking [11,21]. The ACOG committee opinion on cesarean section on maternal request includes a review of research on elective cesarean delivery without labor [11]. Studies reviewed showed that neonatal respiratory risks were elevated among elective cesarean delivery without labor compared with vaginal delivery when delivery occurred before 39 to 40 weeks of gestation. In addition, complications associated with prematurity, such as respiratory symptoms, hypothermia, hypoglycemia, and NICU admissions, were higher among infants delivered by elective cesarean section without labor before 39 weeks of gestation. Considering these complications related to iatrogenic prematurity, ACOG recommends that cesarean delivery on maternal request should not be performed before a gestational age of 39 weeks has been accurately determined unless there is verification of lung maturity [11]. The degree to which cesarean delivery on maternal request is or is not contributing to iatrogenic prematurity is currently unknown.

Weighing the risks

The overall increase in the preterm birth rate and the concurrent increase in medically indicated preterm births have been accompanied by a decrease in stillbirth and perinatal mortality rates [8,9,67]. Preterm-related obstetric intervention is undertaken for maternal indications and suspected fetal compromise. It has been posited that the risk tolerance and threshold for obstetric intervention has decreased with advances in neonatal and obstetric care resulting in increased preterm survival [9]. In addition, obstetric intervention has increased in late preterm gestational ages [9,67]. There are two clinical questions that must be addressed when intervention before term is contemplated. The first regards the necessity for delivery, and the second regards the route of delivery. Information on vital records cannot provide these answers on a case-by-case basis; this information only documents the occurrence of the birth, selected perinatal factors, and route of delivery. Hence, population-based analyses that account for weighing risks are lacking.

Many high-risk pregnancies have benefited from obstetric intervention at 34 to 36 weeks, as suggested by declines in rates of fetal demise during the same gestational period [9]. As such, the increase in medically indicated preterm birth might be positively viewed in light of the reduction of stillbirths and neonatal mortality [8]. However, many improvements in neonatal and maternal management could also explain some of these findings. Considering that neonatal and infant mortality for late preterm births exceeds that of term births [45,68], every effort should be made to prevent unnecessary iatrogenic early birth. Taken together, obstetric interventions at preterm gestation to reduce risks for the mother and fetus need to be optimally balanced with risks associated with preterm birth. This balance becomes even more challenging when growing obstetric malpractice pressures are added to the equation [69].

Future research

Given our findings that the increase in the preterm birth rate occurred primarily among cesarean sections, it is imperative to conduct well-designed adequately powered studies that focus on the underlying reasons for the escalation in preterm birth and cesarean section rates. Additionally, estimates of the proportion of cesarean section deliveries that are not medically or obstetrically indicated need to be determined. Such clinical investigations require access to accurately reported data on maternal and fetal indications resulting in iatrogenic preterm birth. Although many potential indications are currently reported on the birth certificate, they have been shown to be underreported [51–53]. This underscores the need for computerized clinical databases to provide the necessary variables to understand the complex array of risks, benefits, and ultimate management that supported the method of delivery and perinatal outcomes. Furthermore, research is needed on the impact of medical intervention on maternal and neonatal morbidity to optimally balance risks and benefits, and thereby provide additional guidance in difficult obstetric management decisions.

Summary

The increasing trend of delivering at earlier gestational ages has raised concerns of the impact on maternal and infant health. The delicate balance of the risks and benefits associated with continuing a pregnancy versus delivering early remains challenging. Among singleton live births in the United States, the proportion of preterm births increased from 9.7% to 10.7% between 1996 and 2004. The increase in singleton preterm births occurred primarily among those delivered by cesarean section, with the largest percentage increase in late preterm births. For all maternal racial/ethnic groups, singleton cesarean section rates increased for each gestational age group. Singleton cesarean section rates for non-Hispanic black women increased at a faster pace among all preterm gestational age groups compared with non-Hispanic white and Hispanic women. Further research is needed to understand the underlying reasons for the increase in cesarean section deliveries resulting in preterm birth.

References

[1] Davidoff MJ, Dias T, Damus K, et al. Changes in the gestational age distribution among U.S. singleton births: impact on rates of late preterm birth, 1992 to 2002. Semin Perinatol 2006;30(1):8–15.

[2] Institute of Medicine. Section IV. Consequences of preterm birth. In: Behrman RE, Butler AS, editors. Preterm birth: causes, consequences, and prevention. Washington, DC: National Academies Press; 2006. p. 311–45.

[3] Martin JA, Hamilton BE, Sutton PD, et al. Births: final data for 2005. Natl Vital Stat Rep 2007;56(6):1–104.

[4] DeFrances CJ, Hall MJ. 2005 National hospital discharge survey. Adv Data 2007;385:1–19.

[5] March of Dimes/Peristats. National center for health statistics data. Available at: http://www.marchofdimes.com/Peristats. Accessed January 20, 2007.

[6] Slattery MM, Morrison JJ. Preterm delivery. Lancet 2002;360(9344):1489–97.

[7] Callaghan WM, MacDorman MF, Rasmussen SA, et al. The contribution of preterm birth to infant mortality rates in the United States. Pediatrics 2006;118(4):1566–73.

[8] Ananth CV, Joseph KS, Oyelese Y, et al. Trends in preterm birth and perinatal mortality among singletons: United States, 1989 through 2000. Obstet Gynecol 2005;105(5 Pt 1): 1084–91.

[9] Joseph KS, Demissie K, Kramer MS. Obstetric intervention, stillbirth, and preterm birth. Semin Perinatol 2002;26(4):250–9.

[10] American College of Obstetricians and Gynecologists. ACOG practice bulletin 10: induction of labor. Int J Gynaecol Obstet 2000;69(3):283–92.

[11] American College of Obstetricians and Gynecologists. ACOG Committee opinion no. 386 November 2007: cesarean delivery on maternal request. Obstet Gynecol 2007;110(5):1209–12.

[12] MacDorman MF, Mathews TJ, Martin JA, et al. Trends and characteristics of induced labour in the United States, 1989–98. Paediatr Perinat Epidemiol 2002;16(3):263–73.

[13] Placek PJ, Taffel SM. Recent patterns in cesarean delivery in the United States. Obstet Gynecol Clin North Am 1988;15(4):607–27.

[14] Taffel SM, Placek PJ, Moien M, et al. 1989 U.S. cesarean section rate steadies—VBAC rate rises to nearly one in five. Birth 1991;18(2):73–7.

[15] Burrows LJ, Meyn LA, Weber AM. Maternal morbidity associated with vaginal versus cesarean delivery. Obstet Gynecol 2004;103(5 Pt 1):907–12.

[16] Kelleher CJ, Cardozo LD. Caesarean section: a safe operation? J Obstet Gynaecol 1994;14: 86–90.

[17] Wu S, Kocherginsky M, Hibbard JU. Abnormal placentation: twenty-year analysis. Am J Obstet Gynecol 2005;192(5):1458–61.

[18] Villar J, Carroli G, Zavaleta N, et al. Maternal and neonatal individual risks and benefits associated with caesarean delivery: multicentre prospective study. BMJ 2007;335(7628):1025.

[19] Bewley S, Cockburn J. II. The unfacts of 'request' caesarean section. BJOG 2002;109(6): 597–605.

[20] Webb DA, Robbins JM. Mode of delivery and risk of postpartum rehospitalization. JAMA 2003;289(1):46–7.

[21] NIH. NIH State-of-the-Science Conference Statement on cesarean delivery on maternal request. NIH Consens Sci Statements 2006;23(1):1–29.

[22] Liu S, Liston RM, Joseph KS, et al. Maternal mortality and severe morbidity associated with low-risk planned cesarean delivery versus planned vaginal delivery at term. CMAJ 2007; 176(4):455–60.

[23] Declercq E, Barger M, Cabral HJ, et al. Maternal outcomes associated with planned primary cesarean births compared with planned vaginal births. Obstet Gynecol 2007;109(3): 669–77.

[24] Alexander JM, Leveno KJ, Hauth J, et al. Fetal injury associated with cesarean delivery. Obstet Gynecol 2006;108(4):885–90.

[25] Gerten KA, Coonrod DV, Bay RC, et al. Cesarean delivery and respiratory distress syndrome: does labor make a difference? Am J Obstet Gynecol 2005;193(3 Pt 2):1061–4.

[26] Hansen AK, Wisborg K, Uldbjerg N, et al. Risk of respiratory morbidity in term infants delivered by elective caesarean section: cohort study. BMJ 2008;336(7635):85–7.

[27] Nisenblat V, Barak S, Griness OB, et al. Maternal complications associated with multiple cesarean deliveries. Obstet Gynecol 2006;108(1):21–6.

[28] Silver RM, Landon MB, Rouse DJ, et al. Maternal morbidity associated with multiple repeat cesarean deliveries. Obstet Gynecol 2006;107(6):1226–32.

[29] American College of Obstetricians and Gynecologists. ACOG practice bulletin no. 54: vaginal birth after previous cesarean. Obstet Gynecol 2004;104(1):203–12.

[30] American College of Obstetricians and Gynecologists. Vaginal delivery after previous cesarean birth. Number 1—August 1995. Committee on Practice Patterns. American College of Obstetricians and Gynecologists. Int J Gynaecol Obstet 1996;52(1):90–8.

[31] Lydon-Rochelle M, Holt VL, Easterling TR, et al. Risk of uterine rupture during labor among women with a prior cesarean delivery. N Engl J Med 2001;345(1):3–8.

[32] Sachs BP, Kobelin C, Castro MA, et al. The risks of lowering the cesarean-delivery rate. N Engl J Med 1999;340(1):54–7.

[33] Greene MF. Vaginal delivery after cesarean section—is the risk acceptable? N Engl J Med 2001;345(1):54–5.

[34] Menacker F. Trends in cesarean rates for first births and repeat cesarean rates for low-risk women: United States, 1990–2003. Natl Vital Stat Rep 2005;54(4):1–8.

[35] Raju TN. Epidemiology of late preterm (near-term) births. Clin Perinatol 2006;33(4):751–63.

[36] Wang ML, Dorer DJ, Fleming MP, et al. Clinical outcomes of near-term infants. Pediatrics 2004;114(2):372–6.

[37] Sarici SU, Serdar MA, Korkmaz A, et al. Incidence, course, and prediction of hyperbilirubinemia in near-term and term newborns. Pediatrics 2004;113(4):775–80.

[38] Seubert DE, Stetzer BP, Wolfe HM, et al. Delivery of the marginally preterm infant: what are the minor morbidities? Am J Obstet Gynecol 1999;181(5 Pt 1):1087–91.

[39] Engle WA, Tomashek KM, Wallman C. "Late-preterm" infants: a population at risk. Pediatrics 2007;120(6):1390–401.

[40] McIntire DD, Leveno KJ. Neonatal mortality and morbidity rates in late preterm births compared with births at term. Obstet Gynecol 2008;111(1):35–41.

[41] Gilbert WM, Nesbitt TS, Danielsen B. The cost of prematurity: quantification by gestational age and birth weight. Obstet Gynecol 2003;102(3):488–92.

[42] Escobar GJ, Greene JD, Hulac P, et al. Rehospitalisation after birth hospitalisation: patterns among infants of all gestations. Arch Dis Child 2005;90(2):125–31.

[43] Tomashek KM, Shapiro-Mendoza CK, Weiss J, et al. Early discharge among late preterm and term newborns and risk of neonatal morbidity. Semin Perinatol 2006;30(2):61–8.

[44] Mathews TJ, MacDorman MF. Infant mortality statistics from the 2004 period linked birth/infant death data set. Natl Vital Stat Rep 2007;55(14):1–32.

[45] Tomashek KM, Shapiro-Mendoza CK, Davidoff MJ, et al. Differences in mortality between late-preterm and term singleton infants in the United States, 1995–2002. J Pediatr 2007; 151(5):450–6.

[46] Heffner LJ, Elkin E, Fretts RC. Impact of labor induction, gestational age, and maternal age on cesarean delivery rates. Obstet Gynecol 2003;102(2):287–93.

[47] Lydon-Rochelle MT, Holt VL, Nelson JC, et al. Accuracy of reporting maternal in-hospital diagnoses and intrapartum procedures in Washington State linked birth records. Paediatr Perinat Epidemiol 2005;19(6):460–71.

[48] Vahratian A, Buekens P, Alexander GR. State-specific trends in preterm delivery: are rates really declining among non-Hispanic African Americans across the United States? Matern Child Health J 2006;10(1):27–32.

[49] Declercq E, Menacker F, Macdorman M. Maternal risk profiles and the primary cesarean rate in the United States, 1991–2002. Am J Public Health 2006;96(5):867–72.

[50] Bailit JL, Love TE, Mercer B. Rising cesarean rates: are patients sicker? Am J Obstet Gynecol 2004;191(3):800–3.

[51] Parrish KM, Holt VL, Connell FA, et al. Variations in the accuracy of obstetric procedures and diagnoses on birth records in Washington State, 1989. Am J Epidemiol 1993;138(2):119–27.

[52] Piper JM, Mitchel EF Jr, Snowden M, et al. Validation of 1989 Tennessee birth certificates using maternal and newborn hospital records. Am J Epidemiol 1993;137(7):758–68.

[53] Lydon-Rochelle MT, Holt VL, Cardenas V, et al. The reporting of pre-existing maternal medical conditions and complications of pregnancy on birth certificates and in hospital discharge data. Am J Obstet Gynecol 2005;193(1):125–34.

[54] Dietz PM, Callaghan WM, Morrow B, et al. Population-based assessment of the risk of primary cesarean delivery due to excess prepregnancy weight among nulliparous women delivering term infants. Matern Child Health J 2005;9(3):237–44.

[55] Chu SY, Kim SY, Schmid CH, et al. Maternal obesity and risk of cesarean delivery: a meta-analysis. Obes Rev 2007;8(5):385–94.

[56] Guihard P, Blondel B. Trends in risk factors for caesarean sections in France between 1981 and 1995: lessons for reducing the rates in the future. BJOG 2001;108(1):48–55.

[57] LaCoursiere DY, Bloebaum L, Duncan JD, et al. Population-based trends and correlates of maternal overweight and obesity, Utah 1991–2001. Am J Obstet Gynecol 2005;192(3):832–9.

[58] Lu GC, Rouse DJ, DuBard M, et al. The effect of the increasing prevalence of maternal obesity on perinatal morbidity. Am J Obstet Gynecol 2001;185(4):845–9.

[59] Ananth CV, Vintzileos AM. Maternal-fetal conditions necessitating a medical intervention resulting in preterm birth. Am J Obstet Gynecol 2006;195(6):1557–63.

[60] Meis PJ, Michielutte R, Peters TJ, et al. Factors associated with preterm birth in Cardiff, Wales. II. Indicated and spontaneous preterm birth. Am J Obstet Gynecol 1995;173(2): 597–602.

[61] Ananth CV, Vintzileos AM. Epidemiology of preterm birth and its clinical subtypes. J Matern Fetal Neonatal Med 2006;19(12):773–82.

[62] American College of Obstetricians and Gynecologists. ACOG practice bulletin. Diagnosis and management of preeclampsia and eclampsia. Number 33, January 2002. Obstet Gynecol 2002;99(1):159–67.

[63] Hauth JC, Ewell MG, Levine RJ, et al. Pregnancy outcomes in healthy nulliparas who developed hypertension. Calcium for Preeclampsia Prevention Study Group. Obstet Gynecol 2000;95(1):24–8.

[64] Sibai BM. Preeclampsia as a cause of preterm and late preterm (near-term) births. Semin Perinatol 2006;30(1):16–9.

[65] Fuchs K, Wapner R. Elective cesarean section and induction and their impact on late preterm births. Clin Perinatol 2006;33(4):793–801.

[66] McCourt C, Weaver J, Statham H, et al. Elective cesarean section and decision making: a critical review of the literature. Birth 2007;34(1):65–79.

[67] Joseph KS, Allen AC, Dodds L, et al. Causes and consequences of recent increases in preterm birth among twins. Obstet Gynecol 2001;98(1):57–64.

[68] Kramer MS, Demissie K, Yang H, et al. The contribution of mild and moderate preterm birth to infant mortality. Fetal and Infant Health Study Group of the Canadian Perinatal Surveillance System. JAMA 2000;284(7):843–9.

[69] Baicker K, Buckles KS, Chandra A. Geographic variation in the appropriate use of cesarean delivery. Health Aff (Millwood) 2006;25(5):w355–67.

CLINICS IN
PERINATOLOGY

Clin Perinatol 35 (2008) 325–341

Late Preterm Infants, Early Term Infants, and Timing of Elective Deliveries

William A. Engle, MD[a],*,
Michelle A. Kominiarek, MD[b]

[a]Section of Neonatal-Perinatal Pediatrics, Indiana University School of Medicine,
699 West Drive, RR-208, Indianapolis, IN 46202–5119, USA
[b]Division of Maternal Fetal Medicine, Indiana University School of Medicine,
550 North University Boulevard, Room 2440, Indianapolis, IN 46202, USA

Delivery of infants who are physiologically mature and capable of successful transition to the extrauterine environment is an important priority for obstetric practitioners [1]. A corollary of this goal is to avoid iatrogenic complications of prematurity and maternal complications from delivery. It is generally accepted that births should occur at a minimum of 39 weeks' gestation unless earlier delivery occurs spontaneously or because of maternal or fetal medical indications. During the past 15 years in the United States, however, the percentage of infants born before 40 weeks' gestation has dramatically increased and the percentage of infants born after 40 weeks' gestation has decreased [2,3]. The shift in gestational age at birth raises the risk for the birth of physiologically immature infants and associated complications. The purpose of this review is to describe the consequences of birth before physiologic maturity in late preterm and term infants, to identify factors contributing to the decline in gestational age of deliveries in the United States, and to describe strategies to reduce premature delivery of late preterm (34 0/7–36 6/7 weeks' gestation) and early term infants (37 0/7–38 6/7 weeks' gestation) (Fig. 1).

Consequences after birth for late preterm infants and early term infants

During the past decade in the United States, delivery of late preterm infants and infants aged 37 0/7 to 39 6/7 weeks' gestation has increased by 14% and 21%, respectively, whereas births of infants after 40 weeks'

* Corresponding author.
E-mail address: wengle@iupui.edu (W.A. Engle).

0095-5108/08/$ - see front matter © 2008 Elsevier Inc. All rights reserved.
doi:10.1016/j.clp.2008.03.003   *perinatology.theclinics.com*

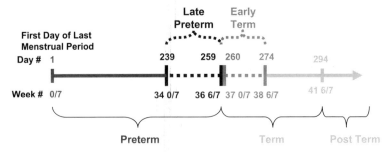

Fig. 1. "Late preterm" and "early term" definitions.

gestation have declined [2]. There are approximately 500,000 preterm births (births before 37 completed weeks of gestation), which account for 12.5% of live births in the United States annually. Of these preterm births, greater than 70% (approximately 350,000 live births) are late preterm. Another 700,000 births (17.5% of live births) occur at 37 and 38 weeks' gestation each year (early term infants) [4]. Both of these groups of infants may experience short-term and long-term consequences associated with premature delivery, whether indicated or elective.

Complications of prematurity in late preterm infants

Late preterm infants are at greater risk than term infants for complications of prematurity [5–9]. During the birth hospitalization, infants born at 34 0/7 to 36 6/7 weeks' gestation compared with term infants experience more difficulties with feeding (32% versus 7%), hypoglycemia (16% versus 5%), jaundice (54% versus 38%), temperature instability (10% versus 0%), apnea (~6% versus < 0.1%), and respiratory distress (29% versus 4%) [7]. Late preterm infants also receive intravenous fluids (27% versus 5%), evaluations for sepsis (37% versus 13%), and mechanical ventilation (3.4% versus 0.9%) more often than their term counterparts. Late preterm infants are 3.5 times more likely to have two or more of these problems than term infants [5]. Because of these medical illnesses and management requirements, many of these infants need specialty care and hospitalizations beyond 5 nights in neonatal intensive care units [8]. Admission for intensive care is inversely proportional to gestational age [10]. In a large health care system, 88% of infants born at 34 weeks' gestation, 12% born at 37 weeks' gestation, and 2.6% born at 38 to 40 weeks' gestation were admitted to an intensive care unit [10]. Duration of hospital stay is also inversely proportional to gestational age [7,10–12].

Hospital readmission and late preterm infants

Late preterm infants who are discharged within the first days after birth are readmitted 1.5 to 3 times more often than term infants [5,10,13]. Rates of readmission to the hospital or an observational stay in late preterm and term infants were 4.3% and 2.7%, respectively, in a large population-based study of singleton infants [14]. The primary reasons for readmission of late preterm infants are hyperbilirubinemia (71%), suspected infection (20%), and feeding difficulty (16%), problems that reflect developing physiologic and metabolic organ functions [5,15]. Several risk factors for readmission of late preterm infants have been identified; these include firstborn or breastfed, maternal labor and delivery complications, recipients of public insurance, and Asian-Pacific Island descent [16]. Because readmission rates are increased in late preterm infants, it is important to focus care and support before discharge on the problems that may present during the first days and weeks at home, such as feeding issues and jaundice. Oral feeding dysfunction may only become apparent after the mother's breast milk supply increases and the infant's oromotor skills are challenged. Furthermore, concentrations of bilirubin, a neural toxin, may peak after discharge from the initial hospitalization in late preterm infants.

Mortality, long-term morbidity, and late preterm infants

Mortality rates beyond the first month after birth are higher in late preterm infants than in term infants [5,17]. Neonatal mortality (deaths among infants 0–27 days' chronologic age) is 4.6 times higher than in term infants (4.1 versus 0.9 per 1000 live births in 2002, respectively) [17,18]. Infant mortality (deaths among infants 0–364 days' chronologic age) has been consistently higher in late preterm infants than in term infants for the past 15 years. In 2002, the infant mortality rate was 7.7 versus 2.5 per 1000 live births in late preterm and term infants, respectively [5,19]. Interestingly, infant mortality is greater in late preterm infants for each of the leading 10 causes of death (Table 1). In addition to an increased risk for mortality, late preterm infants have higher relative rates of developmental handicaps than term infants. Specifically, school performance difficulties and behavioral disabilities, especially attention deficit hyperactivity disorder, are

Table 1
Cause-specific infant mortality rates of late preterm and term infants (per 100,000 live births)

	Late preterm (rank)	Term (rank)
Congenital anomalies	333 (1)	77 (1)
Sudden infant death syndrome	99 (2)	49 (2)
Accidents (unintentional)	38 (3)	21 (3)
Disease of the circulatory system	25 (4)	10 (4)
Intrauterine hypoxia and birth asphyxia	17 (5)	7 (5)
Influenza and pneumonia	12 (6)	5 (7)
Assault (homicide)	12 (7)	6 (6)
Bacterial sepsis of the newborn	11 (8)	3 (9)
Newborn affected by complications of the placenta, cord, or membranes	11 (9)	2 (10)
Atelectasis	10 (10)	0.7 (24)

Table 2
Attention deficit hyperactivity disorder and gestational age

Gestational age (weeks)	Controls n = 20,100	ADHD cases n = 834 (%)	Adjusted relative risk (95% confidence interval)
<34	298	34 (11.4)	2.7 (1.8–4.1)
34–36	544	37 (6.8)	1.7 (1.2–2.5)
37–39	6629	298 (4.5)	1.1 (0.9–1.3)
40–42	12,365	456 (3.7)	Reference
43–44	264	9 (3.4)	1.0 (0.5–2.0)

Data from Linnet KM, Wisborg K, Agerbo E, et al. Gestational age, birth weight, and the risk of hyperkinetic disorder. Arch Dis Child 2006;9:655–60.

more prevalent in late preterm infants (Tables 2 and 3) [20–22]. Such impairments may relate to incomplete brain development after birth in late preterm infants [21]. At birth, the brain mass of late preterm infants is only approximately 70% that of term infants and myelinization is markedly underdeveloped.

Most late preterm infants thrive after birth and have no complications or long-term impairments. Because of the risks for mortality and morbidity associated with birth at 34 0/7 to 36 6/7 weeks' gestation, however, such infants need close monitoring and follow-up. Additional investigations to understand the causes for late preterm births better and efforts to prevent them, if possible, are warranted.

Respiratory morbidities, possible long-term morbidities, and early term infants

In a large retrospective review of the incidence of respiratory distress in term and late preterm infants, 1.9% experienced respiratory distress because of transient tachypnea, respiratory distress syndrome, or persistent pulmonary hypertension of the newborn (Table 4) [23]. A review of studies of term infants found that the incidence of transient tachypnea of the newborn, respiratory distress syndrome, and persistent pulmonary hypertension of the newborn were approximately 3.1%, 0.25%, and 0.17%, respectively

Table 3
School age outcome of healthy late preterm (n = 22,552) versus healthy term (n = 164,628) infants in Florida

Outcome	Age (years)	Relative risk (95% confidence interval)
Developmental delay or disability	0–3	1.46 (1.42–1.50)
Special education	5	1.13 (1.11–1.15)
Grade retention	5	1.11 (1.08–1.14)

Data from Adams-Chapman I. Neurodevelopmental outcome of the late preterm infant. Clin Perinatol 2006;30:947–64; with permission, and Morse SB, Tang Y, Roth J. School-age outcomes of healthy near-term infants (34–37 weeks) versus healthy term infants (38–42 weeks). Pediatr Res 2006;1(Suppl):158.

Table 4
Incidence of respiratory morbidity in late preterm and term infants

	Cesarean section n = 4301 (%)	Vaginal birth n = 21,017 (%)	Combined n = 25,318 (%)	Odds ratio (95% confidence interval) for cesarean section versus vaginal birth
Transient tachypnea of the newborn	151 (3.5)	238 (1.1)	389 (1.5)	3.3 (2.6–3.9)
Respiratory distress syndrome	20 (0.47)	33 (0.16)	53 (0.21)	3.0 (1.6–5.3)
Persistent pulmonary hypertension	17 (0.4)	17 (0.08)	34 (0.13)	4.9 (2.2–8.8)
Total	188 (4.4)	288 (1.4)	476 (1.9)	3.3 (2.7–4.0)

Data from Levine EM, Ghai V, Barton JJ, et al. Mode of delivery and risk of respiratory disease in newborn. Obstet Gynecol 2001;97:440.

(weighted calculation based on one third of infants being born by cesarean delivery) (Table 5) [24]. Considering that 87.5% of the 4 million deliveries annually in the United States occur at term and more than 3% neonates have respiratory disorders after birth, approximately 105,000 newborns are affected, require additional medical interventions, are exposed to complications of intensive care, and, although infrequent, die from their illnesses. Importantly, infants with respiratory distress are temporarily separated from their mothers and families.

According to a retrospective geographically based analysis of 179,701 births, the incidence of severe respiratory distress syndrome in infants aged 34 to 41 weeks' gestation declines with increasing gestational age (Table 6) [25]. Infants born at 37 weeks' gestation have a 3-fold greater rate of respiratory distress syndrome that those born at 38 weeks' gestation, who, in turn, have a 7.5-fold greater rate than infants born at 39 to 41 weeks' gestation. Infants born at 37 to 38 weeks' gestation also have a significantly

Table 5
Incidence of respiratory morbidity in term infants and effect of cesarean section

	Cesarean section	Vaginal birth	Range of odds ratios for cesarean section versus vaginal birth (range)
Transient tachypnea of the newborn	0.9%–12%	0.3%–3%	1.2–2.8
Respiratory distress syndrome	0.2–0.7%	0.1–0.2%	0–7.1
Persistent pulmonary hypertension of the newborn	0.37%	0.08%	4.6

Data from Kirkeby Hansen A, Wisborg K, Uldbjerg N, et al. Elective caesarean section and respiratory morbidity in the term and near-term neonate. Acta Obstet Gynecol Scand 2007;86:392.

Table 6
Respiratory distress syndrome in late preterm and term infants

Gestational age (weeks)	Incidence of respiratory distress syndrome (per 1000 infants)	Relative rate compared with following gestation
34	30	2.1
35	14	2.0
36	7.1	3.9
37	1.8	3.0
38	0.6	7.5
39–41	0.08	Reference

Data from Madar J, Richmond S, Hey E. Surfactant-deficient respiratory distress after elective delivery at 'term.' Acta Paediatr 1999;88:1245.

higher risk for transient tachypnea of the newborn, persistent pulmonary hypertension, hospital stays beyond 5 nights, and diagnoses associated with severe morbidities or death than infants born at 39 weeks' gestation [3,8,9,24–27].

Delivery by cesarean section is an important independent risk factor for respiratory morbidity in term infants. Studies of infants delivered by elective cesarean section have consistently shown that the risk for respiratory distress syndrome and transient tachypnea of the newborn is inversely proportional to gestational age [7,9,24,25,27–30]. Respiratory distress syndrome and transient tachypnea of the newborn is 1.7 times more frequent at 37 weeks' gestation compared with 38 weeks' gestation and 2.4 times as frequent at 38 weeks' gestation compared with 39 weeks' gestation in infants delivered by elective cesarean section [31]. Long-term morbidities in term infants have been inconsistently correlated with birth by cesarean section. Such morbidities include asthma, hay fever, respiratory and food allergies, and diarrhea [32–35].

Factors contributing to increased birth rate of late preterm and early term infants

Birth before fetal maturity contributes to short-term and long-term morbidity and mortality in late preterm and early term infants. Most babies born between 34 and 38 weeks' gestation are delivered prematurely because of maternal or fetal medical indications [2,36]. All categories of live births (spontaneous, associated with premature rupture of membranes, and associated with medical intervention) of infants born at 34 to 36 weeks' gestation and 37 to 39 weeks' gestation increased as a percent of live births between 1992 and 2002. During this same interval, the percent of live births attributed to infants with gestational ages of 40 to 44 weeks declined considerably, whereas births of infants aged less than 32 weeks' gestation remained stable or decreased.

The reasons for the increase in rates of late preterm and early term births are unclear because of a paucity of information [28]. Several disparate factors have been implicated as important influences on these rates [36–40]:

- Increased medical surveillance and interventions
- Inaccurate gestational age assessment during elective deliveries
- Presumption of fetal maturity at 34 weeks' gestation
- Increase in multifetal pregnancies
- Changes in maternal demographics and health
  - Delayed childbearing and increased risk for prematurity
  - Use of assisted reproductive technologies (multifetal pregnancies)
  - Maternal obesity and increased risk for complications associated with premature delivery (eg, preeclampsia, diabetes)
- Maternal autonomy and route and timing of delivery
  - Cesarean or planned induction of labor
    - Indicated: abnormal presentation, abnormal placentation, maternal or fetal conditions (eg, premature rupture of membranes without labor, fetal hydrocephalus)
    - Repeat
    - Without medical indication (induction of labor or cesarean section on maternal request)
  - Fear of fetal and neonatal risks with vaginal delivery
    - Increased rate of stillbirths beginning at 39 weeks' gestation
    - Hypoxic ischemic encephalopathy, brachial plexus, and other birth trauma, especially with breech or other abnormal presentation
  - Fear of fetal and neonatal risks with cesarean delivery
    - Higher rates of mortality, respiratory and other acute morbidity, neonatal intensive care, separation from family, longer hospital stay
  - Fear of maternal risks with vaginal delivery
    - Risk for genital tract, anus, and perineal injury and sexual dysfunction
    - Perception that cesarean delivery is "easier" and "less stressful" than vaginal delivery
    - Fear of the second stage and having to "push the baby out"
  - Fear of maternal risks with cesarean delivery
    - Bladder injury, hemorrhage, death, hysterectomy, intensive care, repeat cesarean section, abnormal placentation in future pregnancies, future fetal loss, poor perception of birth experience, financial costs, repeat hospitalization
  - Maternal willingness to accept risk on behalf of the infant
    - Convenience for mother and family
- Physician practice patterns and risk/benefit determination
  - Convenience
  - Liability

Accuracy of obstetric estimates of gestational age

Estimating the delivery date and gestational age prenatally is inexact because the commonly used methods, Naegle's rule (calculated from the first date of the last menstrual period) and the second trimester sonogram, are both accurate to only within 1 to 2 weeks [41,42]. Naegle's rule depends on the assumptions that a woman's menstrual cycles are regular and occur every 28 days, recall is accurate, and ovulation occurs 14 days after the first day of the last menstrual period. Only approximately 30% of women are in their fertile window 10 to 17 days after the first day of the last menstrual period [43]. Maternal recall is frequently not dependable, menstrual cycles may vary considerably, vaginal bleeding or spotting may occur during the first few cycles after fertilization, and use of oral contraceptives often alters menstrual periodicity. Combined with inherent biologic variability in fetal maturation at any one gestational age, the accuracy of the commonly used prenatal methods to determine fetal gestational age and the estimated date of delivery is limited. If dates associated with artificial reproductive technologies or first trimester ultrasonogram assessments of the gestational sac (appears at ~5 weeks' gestation), appearance of fetal heart rate (appears at ~6 weeks' gestation), or crown-rump length at 6 to 11 weeks' gestation are performed, accuracy of dating may be within 3 to 5 days of the actual gestational age.

Another important factor in accurate determination of fetal gestational age is obesity, which is an epidemic in the United States [40]. Obesity during pregnancy may be associated with fetal macrosomia and inaccurate ultrasonographic estimation of gestational age. Excess weight gain during pregnancy is protective for preterm delivery (adjusted odds ratio = 0.54, 95% confidence interval: 0.52–0.57), although complications of obesity are associated with preterm delivery (gestational diabetes: adjusted odds ratio = 1.28, 95% confidence interval: 1.20–1.36; pregnancy-associated hypertension: odds ratio = 1.82, 95% confidence interval: 1.67–1.98). Oligohydramnios also interferes with the accuracy of ultrasonographic measurements for gestational age, especially in the setting of premature rupture of membranes. Inaccurate estimations of fetal gestational age pose a degree of uncertainty when counseling patients about the optimal route and timing of delivery, especially if elective induction of labor or cesarean delivery is considered.

Obstetric surveillance

Medical surveillance has intensified with advances in obstetric practices. The primary purpose of antenatal testing and intrapartum monitoring is to identify maternal or fetal complications early in the pathophysiologic process when they may be amenable to interventions to prevent progression of maternal illness or fetal compromise. Electronic fetal monitoring and prenatal ultrasonography were used in 85% and 67% of pregnancies, respectively, in 2003 [5]. In contrast, in 1989, electronic fetal monitoring was used in only 68% of pregnancies and prenatal ultrasonography was used in only 48% of pregnancies. Deliveries after interventions, such as labor induction and elective cesarean section, have also increased during the past 10 years [2,44–47]. Increased use of these and other obstetrics tools has resulted in a reduction in stillbirths and perinatal mortality [4]. Conversely, some antenatal tests (eg, nonstress tests, biophysical profile) have low positive predictive values. As such, an abnormal test result may not reflect the true fetal status. Thus, more intensive testing and monitoring may lead to more delivery interventions and, subsequently, contribute to a higher rate of late preterm and early term births.

Multifetal pregnancies

The percent of live births that accompany multifetal pregnancies increased from 2.4% to 3.2% of live births between 1992 and 2002 [44]. This increase in multifetal gestations is partly explained by artificial reproductive technologies and delayed childbearing. The average gestational age of twin births is 35 weeks [38]. The increase in percent of late preterm and early term births is, at least in part, associated with late preterm delivery of multifetal pregnancies. Recurrent preterm delivery is not prevented in multifetal pregnancies by maternal administration of 17 α-hydroxyprogesterone caproate as it is in singleton births [48,49]. Efforts to understand and discover strategies that safely prolong the duration of gestation in multifetal pregnancies are warranted.

Race and ethnicity

Race and ethnicity have an impact on rates of late preterm and early term deliveries [2]. Non-Hispanic white births accounted for the largest percent increase in births between 1992 and 2002 at 35 weeks' gestation (1.7%–2.0% of live births) and at 36 weeks' gestation (3.1%–3.9% of live births) compared with Hispanic and black births. During this same interval, Hispanic births at 34 and 35 weeks' gestation were stable but increased from 3.7% to 4.1% of live births at 36 weeks' gestation. In contrast, the percentage of births of black infants declined at 34 and 35 weeks' gestation but increased slightly at 36 weeks' gestation. Common among non-Hispanic white, Hispanic, and black births was an increase in the percentage of births at 36 weeks' gestation. The reason why the largest percent change occurred in non-Hispanic white births has not been determined. In a separate study, risk factors frequently associated with preterm birth, such as tobacco use and vaginal infections, were not significantly more common in late preterm infants than in term infants [50]. Factors speculated to account for these differences in perinatal outcomes include socioeconomic status, access to health care, and maternal demand for elective delivery.

Fetal maturity and 34 weeks' gestation

In the past, research protocols and practice guidelines implied that 34 weeks' gestation was a surrogate for fetal maturity; therefore, infants

born at or later than 34 weeks' gestation were considered to be at low risk
for morbidity and mortality [1,39,51]. When such protocols and guidelines
were developed, infant mortality in late preterm infants was within 1% of
that of term infants. Since the publication of these guidelines, a growing
body of literature indicates that late preterm and early term infants are at
risk for respiratory, developmental, and behavioral morbidity in addition
to mortality. It is anticipated that future research and guideline revisions
are likely to consider this rapidly growing body of literature about the morbidities that accompany late preterm and early term birth.

Route and timing of delivery

Patients and physicians must weigh the risks and benefits for each delivery
option when deciding about route and timing of delivery. Spontaneous vaginal deliveries account for approximately 60% of all deliveries, and medical
interventions to effect deliveries account for the remaining 40% [2]. Cesarean
delivery is elective for several reasons (eg, repeat, abnormal presentation,
multifetal pregnancy, maternal request without a medical indication) or
necessitated by intrapartum conditions (eg, cephalopelvic disproportion,
nonreassuring fetal heart rate, failed operative forceps or vacuum delivery).

The rates of cesarean deliveries and inductions of labor have increased
dramatically during the past 10 years. Cesarean sections account for approximately one third of deliveries. Although estimates vary considerably
because of insufficient documentation and lack of prospective investigations
[52,53], Menacker and colleagues [52] estimated that 3% to 7% of cesarean
deliveries were performed without a clear medical indication. Other investigators have reported that elective cesarean deliveries account for as many as
18% of cesarean deliveries in the United States [36]. Inductions of labor
occur in approximately 10% to 20% of deliveries, and roughly half are
performed electively [4,36,44–47,54,55]. Because inductions of labor are so
common, small shifts in clinical thresholds to convert to cesarean delivery
may greatly increase the number of cesarean deliveries [46].

The reasons for the increasing trends in elective cesarean deliveries and
labor inductions are complex. Concern about stillbirth, birth trauma, shoulder dystocia, and neonatal encephalopathy with vaginal birth beyond
39 weeks' gestation and willingness of mothers to incur risk on behalf of
their child are important influences when deciding about timing and route
of delivery [4]. Patient fear of vaginal delivery because of perceived discom-
fort and complications (eg, pelvic floor dysfunction with incontinence and
loss of sexual functioning), complications associated with vaginal breech
delivery, subtle changes in medical thresholds for abandoning vaginal delivery and proceeding to intrapartum cesarean delivery, convenience for families and physicians, the decline in the rate of vaginal birth after cesarean
delivery because of the risk for uterine rupture, and liability concerns of
physicians are also likely influences [4,28].

Neonatal and maternal complications after cesarean and vaginal delivery were prospectively evaluated and reported in 97,095 deliveries [28]. Investigators analyzed data from the 2005 World Health Organization survey on maternal and perinatal health. In this large cohort of deliveries, a significantly increased risk for a neonatal intensive care stay of 7 days or more occurred for cesarean delivery, including elective cesarean delivery (odds ratio $= 2.11$, 95% confidence interval: 1.75–2.55) and intrapartum cesarean delivery (odds ratio $= 1.93$, 95% confidence interval: 1.63–2.29). Mortality in infants with a cephalic presentation delivered by elective cesarean section was also increased 1.7-fold. Similarly, mortality in infants with a cephalic presentation delivered by intrapartum cesarean section was increased 2-fold. Cesarean delivery also significantly reduced mortality associated with breech presentation. Although cesarean delivery reduced vaginal injuries (third and fourth degree lacerations and fistula formation), severe maternal morbidity (eg, death, hysterectomy, blood transfusion, intensive care stay) and antibiotic use were increased 2-fold and 5-fold, respectively. The maternal and neonatal outcomes reported in this large population study support findings from other investigators that cesarean delivery is associated with relatively higher rates of neonatal mortality and prolonged neonatal intensive care stay, severe maternal morbidities, and maternal antibiotic use [36,56,57]. In contrast, cesarean delivery has advantages for breech presentations and maternal perineal injury. In 2007, the American College of Obstetricians and Gynecologists described several benefits of planned cesarean delivery compared with intrapartum cesarean or vaginal delivery that included lower rates of postpartum hemorrhage, transfusion, surgical complications, and urinary incontinence in the first year after delivery [57].

Cesarean delivery is associated with a large list of potential complications, most with weak correlations, that favor vaginal delivery [36,53,56]. Examples of complications associated with cesarean delivery include separation from the mother and delayed breastfeeding; higher rates of postpartum fever, infection, pneumonia, and thromboembolic events; organ injury (eg, bladder, ureter, bowel); lower postpartum health status scores; reduced satisfaction with the birth experience; low self-esteem, depression, and psychologic trauma; longer length of hospital stay; additional laboratory and imaging assessment; additional procedural interventions; and higher cost than vaginal deliveries [36,56–59]. Cesarean delivery also has implications for future deliveries [36,53,56]. Uterine rupture during labor occurs at a higher rate in patients who have had a previous cesarean delivery. Abnormal placentation, such as placenta previa and placenta accreta, increased risk for intrapartum hemorrhage and hysterectomy, and more complicated repeat abdominal surgery because of adhesions may further complicate future deliveries. Counseling about these additional risks related to cesarean delivery is important for patients, especially primigravid women who intend to have more children.

Advances in cervical ripening and induction agents, careful selection of patients with a favorable cervix, and labor induction protocols are believed to have reduced the risks related to labor induction. Despite these improvements, debate about the use of elective induction of labor continues [45,46]. It has been argued that the induction process and higher risk for cesarean delivery, exposure to complications of the procedure, longer hospital stays, and higher costs, especially in primigravid patients or patients with an unfavorable cervix, outweigh the psychosocial and convenience benefits in most cases [46].

Reducing iatrogenic late preterm and early term births

If elective cesarean or labor induction is considered before 39 weeks' gestation, the American College of Obstetricians and Gynecologists has recommended fetal pulmonary maturity confirmation, a surrogate for physiologic maturation [1]. If fetal pulmonary maturity is not proved, however, it may be inferred from any of the following criteria:

- Fetal heart tones have been documented for 20 weeks by nonelectronic fetoscope or for 30 weeks by Doppler.
- It has been 36 weeks since a positive serum or urine human chorionic gonadotropin pregnancy test result by a reliable laboratory.
- Ultrasound measurement of the crown-rump length at 6 to 11 weeks of gestation supports a gestational age equal to or greater than 39 weeks.
- Ultrasound measurements at 12 to 20 weeks of gestation support a clinically determined gestational age of 39 weeks or greater.

Adherence to these recommendations is not uniform [60]. Confidence in current methods of fetal gestational age assessment and complications of amniocentesis may deter obstetricians from confirming fetal pulmonary maturity before elective delivery [60]. Accurate gestational age assessment is essential when determining timing of elective delivery. If gestational age estimates vary by even 1 or 2 weeks, elective induction of labor or elective cesarean section may be associated with premature delivery of a late preterm or early term infant. New methods to determine fetal gestational age more accurately, especially during the end of the second trimester and during the third trimester, are needed.

Antenatal corticosteroids have been proved to reduce the severity of respiratory distress syndrome and survival of infants born before 34 weeks' gestation. Investigators have recently reported benefits from fetal corticosteroid exposure in late preterm and early term infants [61,62]. Antenatal betamethasone administration to effect pulmonary maturation before elective delivery reduced the incidence of respiratory morbidity (transient tachypnea and respiratory distress syndrome) by half (relative risk = 0.46, 95% confidence interval: 0.23–0.93) [61]. Patients receiving betamethasone reported more minor complications (flushing, nausea, pain at the injection site, and increased energy) than patients receiving the placebo in this study. In a large retrospective cohort of 1044 infants, antenatal steroids administered to mothers before 34 weeks' gestation who delivered at 34 to 36 weeks' gestation effected significant reductions in respiratory disorders (24.4% versus 81.6%; $P < .0001$) and respiratory distress syndrome (7.5% versus 35.5%; $P < .0001$). In contrast, a meta-analysis of corticosteroids given after 33 weeks' gestation did not show decreased neonatal morbidity; however, the analysis was limited because of small numbers of infants [63]. Confirmation of the efficacy and safety of antenatal corticosteroids before elective deliveries and at 34 to 38 weeks' gestation is needed.

A recently published study of 21,771 late preterm births (34–36 weeks) occurring over an 18-year period at a single university-based hospital confirmed the increased neonatal morbidity at these gestational ages compared with term births [9]. Eighty percent of these births were attributed to idiopathic preterm labor or premature rupture of membranes. The remaining deliveries were associated with hypertension, placental accidents, fetal problems, and maternal medical problems. It is unknown whether elective deliveries without a medical indication contributed to any of the deliveries in this study because such information was not reported [9]. Details about strategies that may be altered to prolong a pregnancy, such as expectant management of premature rupture of membranes, were also not reported. Furthermore, in non–university-based hospitals, the reasons for elective labor inductions and cesarean deliveries in late preterm infants have not been reported. Thus, additional information is necessary to determine whether there are specific medical interventions or strategies that may reduce the incidence of late preterm and early term births.

Few studies have addressed the benefits of expectant management of premature rupture of membranes at greater than 34 weeks, and two older studies have not shown a benefit [64,65]. A meta-analysis of planned early birth (using oxytocin or prostaglandin) versus expectant management for prelabor premature rupture of membranes in patients at 37 weeks' gestation or greater found no difference in the need for cesarean or operative delivery or neonatal infection [66]. Maternal infection and the proportion of infants admitted to neonatal intensive care units were significantly reduced in the planned early delivery group. These results were unexpected and suggest that planned early birth has advantages over expectant management, at least in infants greater than or equal to 37 weeks' gestation. Better understanding of the outcomes of mothers and infants born at each gestation between 34 and 38 weeks after prelabor premature rupture of membranes is needed to focus efforts to prevent premature delivery.

Iatrogenic late preterm and early term births can be reduced by adherence to guidelines for determining gestational age and elective deliveries (inductions and cesarean sections). Early prenatal care, which should be encouraged, optimizes the opportunities to assess gestational age most accurately, and thus to plan timing and route of delivery. Women requesting cesarean delivery are likely to benefit from a thorough discussion of the advantages and disadvantages of cesarean and vaginal births for the fetus, newborn infant, and woman. If maternal fears of pain, fetal complications, or maternal morbidities with vaginal delivery are the primary reasons to request cesarean delivery, education and counseling about such fears are recommended [56]. Furthermore, the safety and efficacy of alternative management strategies to increase pulmonary maturity or prolong pregnancy, such as maternal corticosteroid administration beyond 34 weeks' gestation and expectant management for premature rupture of membranes without labor, merit additional study.

Summary

1. Late preterm and early term infants are at greater risk than term infants for acute and long-term complications of premature birth.
2. The rates of late preterm and early term births are increasing.
3. Causes for the increase in rates of late preterm and early term infants are unclear. Factors that are hypothesized to be associated with the increase in rates include the following:
   - Increased surveillance and medical interventions
   - Inaccurate gestational age estimates
   - Presumption of fetal maturity at 34 weeks' gestation
   - Changes in maternal demographics and health
   - Increased rates of elective cesarean sections and inductions of labor
   - Maternal and physician concerns about complications of vaginal delivery and subtle changes in medical thresholds for cesarean birth
   - Willingness of mothers to incur risk on behalf of their child
4. The route and timing of delivery of late preterm and early term newborn infants have important implications for short-term and long-term neonatal outcomes.
5. The risks and benefits for spontaneous vaginal delivery, planned induction of labor, or elective cesarean section for mother and infant should be carefully considered by mothers, families, and physicians when determining the optimal timing and route of delivery.
6. Our understanding of the maternal, fetal, neonatal, and long-term outcomes and causes of late preterm and early term births is incomplete.
7. Research is needed to increase our understanding of maternal and infant outcomes of infants born at 34 to 38 weeks' gestation, to determine the efficacy and safety of strategies to optimize these outcomes, and to develop interventions that effect physiologic maturation of the fetus when premature delivery is necessary or elective.

References

[1] Assessment of fetal lung maturity. Practice bulletin number 230. American College of Obstetricians and Gynecologists November 1996.

[2] Davidoff MJ, Dias T, Damus K, et al. Changes in the gestational age distribution among US singleton births; impact on rates of late preterm birth, 1992 to 2002. Semin Perinatol 2006;30: 8–15.

[3] Miesnik SR, Reale BJ. A review of issues surrounding medically elective cesarean delivery. J Obstet Gynecol Neonatal Nurs 2007;36(6):605–15.

[4] Hankins GDV, Clark S, Munn MB. Cesarean section on request at 39 weeks: impact on shoulder dystocia, fetal trauma, neonatal encephalopathy, and intrauterine fetal demise. Semin Perinatol 2006;30:276–87.

[5] Engle WA, Tomashek KM, Wallman C, and the Committee on Fetus and Newborn. "Late-preterm" infants: a population at risk. A clinical report. Pediatrics 2007;120(6): 1390–401.

[6] Engle WA. A recommendation for the definition of "late-preterm" (near-term) and the birth weight-gestational age classification system. Semin Perinatol 2006;30(1):2–7.

[7] Wang ML, Dorer DJ, Fleming M, et al. Clinical outcomes of near-term infants. Pediatrics 2004;114:372–6.

[8] Shapiro-Mendoza CK, Tomashek KM, Kotelchuck M, et al. Effect of late preterm birth and maternal medical conditions on newborn morbidity risk. Pediatrics 2008;121:e223–32. 10.1542/peds.2006-3629.

[9] McIntire DD, Leveno KJ. Neonatal mortality and morbidity rates in late preterm births compared with births at term. Obstet Gynecol 2008;111:35–41.

[10] Escobar GJ, Greene JD, Hulac P, et al. Rehospitalization after birth hospitalization: patterns among infants of all gestations. Arch Dis Child 2005;90:125–31.

[11] Rubaltelli FF, Bonafe L, Tangucci M, et al. Epidemiology of neonatal acute respiratory disorders. Biol Neonate 1998;74:7–15.

[12] Gilbert WM, Nesbitt TS, Danielsen B. The cost of prematurity: quantification by gestational age and birth weight. Obstet Gynecol 2003;102:488–92.

[13] Oddie SJ, Hammal D, Richmond S, et al. Early discharge and readmission to hospital in the first month of life in the Northern Region of the UK during 1998: a case cohort study. Arch Dis Child 2005;90:119–24.

[14] Tomashek KM, Shapiro-Mendoza CK, Weiss J, et al. Early discharge among late preterm and term newborns and risk of neonatal mortality. Semin Perinatol 2006;30:61–8.

[15] Escobar GJ, Joffe S, Gardner MN, et al. Rehospitalization in the first two weeks after discharge from the neonatal intensive care unit. Pediatrics 1999;104(1). Available at: www.pediatrics.org/cgi/content/full/104/1/e2. Accessed April 9, 2008.

[16] Shapiro-Mendoza CK, Tomashek KM, Kotelchuck M, et al. Risk factors for neonatal morbidity and mortality among "healthy" late preterm newborns. Semin Perinatol 2006; 30:54–60.

[17] Kramer MS, Demissie K, Yand H, et al. The contribution of mild and moderate preterm birth to infant mortality. Fetal and Infant Health Study Group of the Canadian Perinatal Surveillance System. JAMA 2000;284:843–9.

[18] Martin JA, Hamilton BE, Sutton PD, et al. Births: final data for 2002. Natl Vital Stat Rep 2003;52:1–114.

[19] Tomashek KM, Shapiro-Mendoza CK, Davidoff MJ, et al. Differences in mortality between late-preterm and term singleton infants in the United States; 1995–2002. J Pediatr 2007;151: 450–6.

[20] Linnet KM, Wisborg K, Agerbo E, et al. Gestational age, birth weight, and the risk of hyperkinetic disorder. Arch Dis Child 2006;9:655–60.

[21] Adams-Chapman I. Neurodevelopmental outcome of the late preterm infant. Clin Perinatol 2006;30:947–64.

[22] Morse SB, Tang Y, Roth J. School-age outcomes of healthy near-term infants (34–37 weeks) versus healthy term infants (38–42 weeks). Pediatr Res 2006;1(Suppl):158.

[23] Levine EM, Ghai V, Barton JJ, et al. Mode of delivery and risk of respiratory disease in newborn. Obstet Gynecol 2001;97:439–42.

[24] Kirkeby Hansen A, Wisborg K, Uldbjerg N, et al. Elective caesarean section and respiratory morbidity in the term and near-term neonate. Acta Obstet Gynecol 2007;86:389–94.

[25] Madar J, Richmond S, Hey E. Surfactant-deficient respiratory distress after elective delivery at 'term.' Acta Paediatr 1999;88:1244–8.

[26] Jain L, Golde G. Respiratory transition in infants delivered by cesarean section. Semin Perinatol 2006;30:296–304.

[27] Sutton L, Sayer GP, Bajuk B, et al. Do very sick neonates born at term have antenatal risks? 2. Infants ventilated primarily for lung disease. Acta Obstet Gynecol Scand 2001; 80:917–25.

[28] Villar J, Carroli C, Zavaleta N, et al. Maternal and neonatal individual risks and benefits associated with caesarean delivery: multicenter prospective study. BMJ 2007;335:1025–36. 10.1136/bmj.39363.706956.55.

[29] Zanardo V, Simbi A, Franzoi M, et al. Neonatal respiratory morbidity risk and mode of delivery at term: influence of timing of elective caesarean delivery. Acta Paediatr 2004;93: 643–7.

[30] Yamazaki H, Torigoe K, Numata O, et al. Neonatal clinical outcome after elective cesarean section before the onset of labor at the 37th and 38th week of gestation. Pediatr Int 2003;4: 379–82.

[31] Morrison JJ, Rennie JM, Milton PJ. Neonatal respiratory morbidity and mode of delivery after term: influence of timing of elective caesarean section. J Obstet Gynaecol 1995; 102(2):101–6.

[32] Salam MT, Margolis HG, McConnell R, et al. Mode of delivery is associated with asthma and allergy occurrences in children. Ann Epidemiol 2006;16:341–6.

[33] Werner A, Ramlau-Hansen CH, Jeppesen SK, et al. Caesarean delivery and risk of developing asthma in the offspring. Acta Paediatr 2006;96:595–9.

[34] Renz-Polseer H, David MR, Buist AS, et al. Caesarean section delivery and the risk of allergic disorders in childhood. Clin Exp Allergy 2005;35:1466–72.

[35] Ribley JS, Smith JM, Redding GJ, et al. Childhood asthma hospitalization risk after cesarean delivery in former term and premature infants. Ann Allergy Asthma Immunol 2005;94(2):228–33.

[36] Fuchs K, Wagner R. Elective cesarean section and induction and their impact on late preterm births. Clin Perinatol 2006;33(4):793–801.

[37] Raju TNK. Epidemiology of late preterm (near-term) births. Clin Perinatol 2006;33:751–63.

[38] Lee YM, Cleary-Goldman J, D'Alton ME. The impact of multiple gestations on late preterm (near-term) births. Clin Perinatol 2006;33(4):777–92.

[39] Antenatal corticosteroid therapy for fetal maturation. ACOG Committee opinion number 273. American College of Obstetricians and Gynecologists May 2002.

[40] Rosenberg TJ, Garber S, Lipkind H, et al. Maternal obesity and diabetes as risk factors for adverse pregnancy outcomes: differences among 4 racial/ethnic groups. Am J Public Health 2005;95:1545–51.

[41] Filley RA, Hadlock FP. Sonographic determination of gestational age. In: Callen PW, editor. Ultrasonography in obstetrics and gynecology. 4th edition. Philadelphia: WB Saunders; 2000. p. 146–70.

[42] Laing FC, Frates MC. Ultrasound evaluation during the first trimester of pregnancy. In: Callen PW, editor. Ultrasonography in obstetrics and gynecology. 4th edition. Philadelphia: WB Saunders; 2000. p. 105–44.

[43] Wilcox AJ, Dunson D, Baird DD. The timing of the "fertile window" in the menstrual cycle: day specific estimates from a prospective study. BMJ 2000;321:1259–62.

[44] Martin JA, Hamilton BE, Sutton PD, et al. Births: final data for 2003. Natl Vital Stat Rep 2005;54(2):1–116.

[45] Grobman WA. Elective induction: when? Ever? Clin Obstet Gynecol 2007;50(2):537–46.

[46] Moore LE, Rayburn WF. Elective induction of labor. Clin Obstet Gynecol 2006;49(3): 698–704.

[47] DeFrances CJ, Hall MJ. 2005 National Hospital Discharge Survey. Advanced data from vital and health statistics; number 385. Hyattsville (MD): National Center for Health Statistics; 2007.

[48] Meis PJ, Klebanoff M, Thom E, et al. Prevention of recurrent preterm delivery by 17 alpha-hydroxyprogesterone caproate. N Engl J Med 2003;348(24):2379–85.

[49] Rouse DJ, Caritis SN, Peaceman AM, et al. A trial of 17 alpha-hydroxyprogesterone caproate to prevent prematurity in twins. N Engl J Med 2007;354:454–61.

[50] Selo-Ojeme DO, Tewari R. Late preterm (32–36 weeks) birth in a North London hospital. J Obstet Gynaecol 2006;26(7):624–6.

[51] Management of preterm labor. Practice bulletin number 43. American College of Obstetricians and Gynecologists May 2003.

[52] Menacker F, Declercq E, Macdorman MF. Cesarean delivery: background, trends, and epidemiology. Semin Perinatol 2006;30(5):235–41.

[53] NIH State-of-the-Science Conference Statement on cesarean delivery on maternal request. NIH Consens State Sci Statements 2006;23(1):1–29.

[54] Rayburn WF, Zhang J. Rising rates of labor induction: present concerns and future strategies. Obstet Gynecol 2002;100:164–7.

[55] Hankins GD, Longo M. The role of stillbirth prevention and later preterm (near-term) births. Semin Perinatol 2006;30:20–3.

[56] American College of Obstetricians and Gynecologists. Cesarean delivery on maternal request. ACOG Committee opinion number 394. Obstet Gynecol 2007;110:1510–4.

[57] Wax JR, Cartin A, Pinette MG, et al. Patient choice cesarean: an evidence-based review. Obstet Gynecol Surv 2004;59:601–16.

[58] Rice Simpson K, Thorman KE. Obstetric "conveniences," elective induction of labor, cesarean birth on demand, and other potentially unnecessary interventions. J Perinat Neonatal Nurs 2005;19:134–44.

[59] Kaufman KE, Bailit JL, Grobman W. Elective induction: an analysis of economic and health consequences. Am J Obstet Gynecol 2002;18:858–63.

[60] Laye MR, Dellinger EH. Timing of scheduled cesarean delivery in patients on a teaching versus private service: adherence to American College of Obstetricians and Gynecologists guidelines and neonatal outcomes. Am J Obstet Gynecol 2006;195:577–84.

[61] Stutchfield P, Whitaker R, Russell I, Antenatal Steroids for Term Elective Caesarean Section (ASTECS) Research Team. Antenatal betamethasone and incidence of neonatal respiratory distress after elective caesarean section: pragmatic randomized trial. BMJ 2005;331(7518): 662.

[62] Ventolini G, Neiger R, Mathews L, et al. Incidence of respiratory disorders in neonates born between 34 and 36 weeks of gestation following exposure to antenatal corticosteroids between 24 and 34 weeks of gestation. Am J Perinatol 2007;10.1055/s-2007-1022470.

[63] Roberts D, Dalziel S. Antenatal corticosteroids for accelerating fetal lung maturation for women at risk of preterm birth. Cochrane Database Syst Rev 2006;(3):CD004454.

[64] Naef RW, Albert JR, Ross EL, et al. Premature rupture of membranes at 34 to 37 weeks' gestation: aggressive versus conservative management. Am J Obstet Gynecol 1998;178: 126–30.

[65] Mercer BM, Crocker LG, Boe NM, et al. Induction versus expectant management in premature rupture of the membranes with mature amniotic fluid at 32 to 36 weeks: a randomized trial. Am J Obstet Gynecol 1993;169:775–82.

[66] Dare MR, Middleton P, Crowther CA, et al. Planned early birth versus expectant management (waiting) for prelabour rupture of membranes at term (37 weeks or more). Cochrane Database Syst Rev 2006;(1):CD005302. 10.1002/14651858.CD005302.pub2.

ELSEVIER
SAUNDERS

CLINICS IN
PERINATOLOGY

Clin Perinatol 35 (2008) 343–360

The Influence of Obstetric Practices on Late Prematurity

Karin Fuchs, MD*, Cynthia Gyamfi, MD

Division of Maternal and Fetal Medicine, Columbia University Medical Center, 622 West 168th Street, New York, NY 10032, USA

Although public attention is frequently drawn to preterm births occurring at the limits of viability, late preterm births—defined as those occurring between 34 weeks 0 days and 36 weeks 6 days—account for most preterm births in the United States [1]. In 2005, the preterm birth rate reached an all-time high of 12.7% [2]. Although the number of preterm births occurring at less than 32 weeks has decreased since 1990, the proportion of infants delivered in the late preterm period has increased 25% over the same period [1,2]. By 2005, late preterm births accounted for more than 8% of all singleton births in the United States [2]. Data from the US National Center for Health Statistics demonstrate that 74% of preterm singleton deliveries in the United States occur in the late preterm period [1].

As the frequency of late preterm birth has increased, new attention has been focused on the outcomes of late preterm infants. Late preterm infants are known to experience significant short-term complications, including respiratory morbidity [3,4], feeding difficulties [5], hypothermia [6], hypoglycemia [6], and hyperbilirubinemia [7]. Numerous studies have shown that late preterm infants face not only increased morbidity but increased mortality when compared with their term counterparts [3]. In addition, long-term sequelae of late preterm birth are becoming evident, with studies showing an increased rate of long-term behavioral and developmental morbidities [8,9].

Despite mounting evidence regarding the increased frequency of late preterm births and the increased morbidity faced by these infants, the etiology of the increased rate of late preterm birth is poorly understood. Unfortunately, there are few objective data to explain this trend definitively. The increased rate of late preterm birth is likely multifactorial in etiology, with

* Corresponding author. Division of Maternal Fetal Medicine, Columbia University Medical Center, 622 West 168th Street, PH 16, New York, NY 10032.
  E-mail address: kmf2121@columbia.edu (K. Fuchs).

0095-5108/08/$ - see front matter © 2008 Elsevier Inc. All rights reserved.
doi:10.1016/j.clp.2008.03.004
perinatology.theclinics.com

a proportion of late preterm births stemming from an increased rate of spontaneous preterm births and others resulting from an increased incidence of iatrogenic interventions in the late preterm period. Many standard obstetric practices call for specific interventions when pregnancy complications arise between 34 and 37 weeks of gestation, and these indicated interventions may lead to an increased incidence of late preterm birth. In this article, the authors review the standard management of several maternal and fetal complications of pregnancy and examine the effect these practices may have on the late preterm birth rate.

Management of pregnancy complications: general principles

When complications arise in pregnancy, physicians must assess the risks for continuing the pregnancy with the risks associated with immediate delivery. Preterm birth—whether spontaneous or indicated—carries with it the risk for significant neonatal morbidity and mortality. Accordingly, certain complications are expectantly managed with the goal of allowing the pregnancy to continue to a more advanced gestational age at which delivery carries less risk for prematurity-related morbidity to the neonate. Expectant management of some complications, however, may result in such significant maternal or fetal morbidity that expeditious delivery is indicated at any gestational age.

Because of the significant prematurity-related complications associated with preterm delivery, most obstetric efforts are directed at prolonging pregnancy and expectantly managing pregnancy complications that arise early in gestation. As gestation progresses, however, the balance shifts in favor of delivery as the risk for prematurity-related complications decreases. Because the survival rate of infants born at or beyond 34 weeks is essentially equivalent to that of those born at term [10], 34 completed weeks of gestation has become a threshold at which obstetric management routinely changes. Beyond 34 weeks, most efforts are no longer directed at prolonging pregnancy and the threshold to deliver becomes far lower when pregnancy complications develop in the late preterm period.

Similarly, most research on the use of antenatal corticosteroids (ACS) has focused on the benefit of ACS administration before 34 weeks of gestation, and few studies have investigated the role of ACS administration at later gestational ages. Given the proved benefit of ACS administration in infants delivered before 34 weeks and the relatively low mortality associated with late preterm birth, the National Institutes of Health Consensus Development Conference on Antenatal Steroids in 1994 and the American College of Obstetricians and Gynecologists (ACOG) recommend that all women at risk for preterm delivery between 24 and 34 weeks of gestation should be considered candidates for ACS treatment [11,12]. Despite data suggesting that administration of ACSs may also decrease neonatal respiratory morbidity associated with deliveries at term [13], there remain no published guidelines in the United States calling for the administration of ACSs to promote fetal lung maturity beyond 34 weeks.

Spontaneous late preterm birth

Spontaneous preterm labor

Preterm labor (PTL)—defined as regular uterine contractions leading to progressive cervical dilation before 37 weeks of gestation—is the most common cause of antepartum admission [14] and precedes up to 50% of preterm births [15]. Among late preterm births, spontaneous PTL accounts for a similar proportion of deliveries. In a recent study by McIntire and Leveno [16], approximately 45% of late preterm births at a single institution were attributed to idiopathic PTL. National data suggest that more than 7% of deliveries resulting from PTL occurred in the late preterm period [1].

Despite the relative frequency of PTL, the pathogenesis of PTL is not well understood. Although some theorize that PTL may represent early activation of the normal labor process, some evidence suggests that PTL may result from a pathologic mechanism [17]. Risk factors for PTL include African-American race, smoking, poor weight gain or low body mass index (BMI), low socioeconomic status, multiple gestations, short cervix, vaginal bleeding, and previous preterm delivery [17,18]. According to Practice Bulletin Number 43, entitled "Management of Preterm Labor," published by the ACOG in May 2003 [18], standard management of PTL should involve the use of tocolysis and glucocorticoids up to 34 weeks of gestation. Restriction of physical activity, bedrest, and hydration have not been shown to decrease preterm birth rates and are not recommended in the treatment of PTL [17,18].

Tocolytics, such as magnesium, calcium channel blockers, nonsteroidal anti-inflammatory drugs (NSAIDs), and β-mimetics, are commonly used to reduce the frequency and intensity of uterine contractions, but the benefit of tocolytic therapy seems to be limited. Although tocolytics may successfully ameliorate uterine contractions, tocolysis has not been shown to prevent preterm delivery or decrease perinatal mortality [17,19]. At best, tocolytic therapy may prolong pregnancy for a short period and may delay delivery so as to allow administration of ACSs. Although the ACOG acknowledges that "the upper limit of gestational age for the use of tocolytic drugs may be a function of the neonatal treatment capabilities in the hospital where the clinician practices" [18], antenatal steroids are only recommended for women at risk for preterm delivery before 34 weeks of gestation [11,12]. Accordingly, because the benefit of tocolytics seems to be limited to prolonging pregnancy to allow for administration of ACSs and because ACSs are only administered until 34 weeks of gestation, there is currently no recommendation supporting the routine use of tocolysis beyond 34 weeks of gestation. By not recommending a trial of tocolysis to arrest PTL that occurs beyond 34 weeks, current management strategies may passively contribute to an increase in the late preterm birth rate. Future research should address the risks and benefits associated with late preterm tocolysis and its potential role in decreasing the incidence of late preterm birth.

Although the long-term use of maintenance tocolysis in patients who have arrested PTL or persistent preterm contractions is controversial, recent evidence has emerged showing that cessation of maintenance tocolysis in the late preterm period is associated with an increased risk for late preterm delivery. In a series of more than 5000 women receiving continuous subcutaneous infusion of terbutaline for the management of PTL, Rebarber and colleagues [20] noted a significantly increased risk for late preterm delivery among patients discontinuing tocolysis between 34 and 36 weeks of gestation. In this study, 72% of women discontinuing their terbutaline infusion at 34 weeks delivered before 37 weeks as compared with 62% of those discontinuing treatment at 35 weeks and 43% at 36 weeks ($P < .05$) [20].

Progesterone supplementation has been shown to reduce the risk for recurrent preterm delivery significantly. In a landmark randomized placebo-controlled study, Meis and colleagues [21] noted that when women with a history of a spontaneous preterm delivery were treated with weekly injections of 17-α-hydroxy-progesterone-acetate (17-OHP) from 16 to 36 weeks of gestation, the risk for recurrent preterm birth was significantly decreased compared with controls. Similarly, Fonseca and colleagues [22] showed that daily treatment with vaginal progesterone suppositories similarly led to a decreased rate of recurrent preterm delivery in high-risk women. Although prophylactic administration of 17-OHP has not been shown to prevent preterm delivery in multiple gestations [23], progesterone supplementation has been shown to reduce the risk for preterm birth in women with a short cervix [24]. Ongoing investigation into the potential role of progesterone in the treatment of active PTL and provider education to encourage the appropriate use of 17-OHP in select populations of high-risk women can be expected to reduce rates of preterm birth, including those occurring in the late preterm period.

Preterm premature rupture of membranes

Premature rupture of membranes (PROM) is defined as the spontaneous rupture of fetal membranes before the onset of labor; preterm premature rupture of membranes (PPROM) refers to rupture of membranes before 37 weeks of gestation. PPROM occurs in 3% of all pregnancies and is responsible for 30% of all preterm deliveries [25]. With regard to late preterm birth, national data demonstrate that more than 20% of cases of PPROM in 2002 occurred in late preterm pregnancies [1]. McIntire and Leveno [16] noted that 35% of late preterm births occurring at their institution between 1988 and 2005 resulted from PPROM. PPROM occurs for a variety of reasons, and risk factors associated with PPROM are similar to those associated with spontaneous PTL [26].

The management of PPROM remains controversial, and depends on the gestational age at PPROM and on maternal and fetal status at the time of rupture. Although PPROM may be associated with intrauterine infection and cord compression, in the absence of evidence of maternal or fetal compromise, expectant management is generally recommended before 34 weeks [26]. According to the ACOG's practice bulletin on "Premature Rupture of Membranes" [26], patients who have PPROM between 24 and 34 weeks of gestation should be managed expectantly and treated with a single course of ACSs to promote fetal lung maturity and prophylactic antibiotics to prolong latency. Use of tocolysis for contractions associated with PPROM has not been shown to result in increased latency [27], and tocolytics, if administered, are usually restricted to short-term use while ACSs are being administered. Evidence of chorioamnionitis, active labor with advanced cervical dilation, or fetal compromise is an indication for prompt delivery at any gestational age to prevent additional neonatal morbidity [25,26]. Similarly, delivery is recommended when PPROM occurs after 34 weeks, or if fetal lung maturity can be demonstrated through amniotic fluid testing between 32 and 34 weeks of gestation [26]. Patients who have a history of PPROM in a prior pregnancy should be treated with progesterone in subsequent pregnancies to decrease the risk for recurrent preterm birth [28].

The recommendation to deliver patients who have PPROM beyond 34 weeks is driven not only by the fact that there are currently no recommendations for administration of antenatal corticosteroids (ACS) in the late preterm period but because expectant management of PPROM beyond 34 weeks of gestation is associated with an increased risk for chorioamnionitis, increased risk for prolonged maternal hospital stay, and decreased umbilical cord pH at delivery [29]. Nevertheless, it should be noted that this report of adverse outcomes associated with expectant management of PPROM beyond 34 weeks was published before prophylactic antibiotics became the mainstay of therapy. Because prophylactic antibiotics have been shown to increase the time to delivery [25] without increasing the risk for maternal or neonatal infection, might it be possible to manage patients who have PPROM expectantly if they remain stable beyond 34 weeks? Is there a role for prophylactic antibiotics and expectant management of PPROM that occurs in the late preterm period?

Maternal complications

Hypertensive disorders: gestational hypertension and preeclampsia

Hypertensive disorders are the most common medical complication of pregnancy and are estimated to affect 6% to 10% of all pregnancies [30]. Gestational hypertension (gHTN) is diagnosed as new finding of a systolic blood pressure (BP) of at least 140 mm Hg or a diastolic BP of at least 90 mm Hg on at least two occasions at least 6 hours apart after the 20 week of gestation in women known to be previously normotensive. Preeclampsia (PEC) is defined as the finding of hypertension with new-onset proteinuria. Severe PEC is defined by the presence of sustained elevations in systolic BP to at least 160 mm Hg or in diastolic BP to at least 110 mm Hg for at least 6 hours or by neurologic symptoms or evidence of end organ damage (renal dysfunction, transaminitis, or placental insufficiency). Young nulliparous women are at increased risk for developing hypertensive disorders in pregnancy, as are women carrying multifetal gestations; women with a history of PEC in a prior pregnancy; and women with underlying chronic hypertension (cHTN), diabetes, renal disease, or thrombophilias [31–34].

Management of gHTN and PEC depends on the gestational age at the time of diagnosis and on maternal and fetal status. Definitive treatment calls for delivery, but the decision to deliver for maternal benefit must be weighed against the fetal risks associated with preterm delivery and the maternal and fetal risks for continued expectant management. Given the significant morbidity and mortality associated with preterm delivery, expectant management is generally recommended when gHTN or mild PEC is diagnosed before term. For gHTN or PEC diagnosed before 34 weeks, management usually consists of close maternal and fetal surveillance with serial laboratory studies and fetal testing in addition to administration of ACSs [30,35]. Expert opinion generally allows for continued expectant management of mild disease until term, whereas preterm delivery is often justified when severe disease is present. Delivery is also recommended at any gestational age if there is acute evidence of maternal distress or fetal compromise with non-reassuring fetal heart tracings (NRFHT) [30]. Fortunately, adverse outcomes are rarely associated with expectant management of mild PEC until 37 weeks, and delaying delivery offers significant fetal benefit by decreasing the risk for prematurity-related morbidity (Table 1) [36].

Clearly, recommendations calling for delivery of women with severe PEC beyond 34 weeks would lead to an increased incidence of late preterm birth among women with severe PEC. Data suggest that women with gHTN and mild PEC are also more likely to be delivered in the late preterm period,

Table 1
Risks for expectant management of preeclampsia between 35 and 37 weeks of gestation

	Mild PEC	Severe PEC
Eclampsia	0.5%	1%–2%
HELLP	2%–3%	6%–10%
Abruption	1%–2%	2%–4%
Pulmonary edema	<1%	2%–4%
IUGR	10%–12%	15%–20%
IUFD	0.5%	1%

eviations: HELLP, Hemolysis, Elevated Liver Enzymes, Low Platelets; IUFD, intra-
ʾl demise; IUGR, intrauterine growth retardation.
ʾ Sibai BM. Preeclampsia as a cause of preterm and later preterm (near-term)
ʾrinatol 2006;30:17.

however [36]. Reported rates of late preterm birth range from 4% to 6% among women with gHTN [32,37,38], from 10% to 11% among women with PEC [32,39], and up to 22% in women with recurrent PEC [39,40]. Unfortunately, the etiology of the late preterm births among women is unknown. Available data do not differentiate iatrogenic deliveries for hypertensive disorders from those deliveries that may result from other causes, such as spontaneous PTL or PPROM [36]. Further research is required to determine the etiology and possible prevention of these late preterm births among women with mild hypertensive disorders.

Previous cesarean delivery

Over the past 4 decades, the cesarean section rate in the United States has increased dramatically to an all-time high of greater than 30% in 2005 [2]. Although the rate of vaginal birth after cesarean section (VBAC) increased through the 1980s to a peak in the mid-1990s, the VBAC rate has decreased since and reached an all-time low of 10.6% in 2003 [41]. As the rate of elective repeat cesarean sections has increased, there has been an increased opportunity for iatrogenic late preterm birth.

To avoid iatrogenic prematurity at the time of elective repeat cesarean delivery, the ACOG states that elective delivery should not be scheduled before 39 weeks of gestation [42]. If elective repeat cesarean sections are performed at 39 weeks of gestation according to ACOG's recommendations, they should have a minimal impact on the increasing rate of late preterm birth. Because of the inherent inaccuracy of pregnancy dating with margins of error of up to 3 weeks in the third trimester, however, elective cesarean section performed at "presumed term" might inadvertently contribute to the increasing incidence of late preterm birth. Because of the inaccuracy of pregnancy dating, specific criteria have been outlined to ensure that a pregnancy can be considered to be at term (Box 1) [42]. If a pregnancy cannot be definitively dated by the criteria outlined by the ACOG, it is recommended that fetal lung maturity be demonstrated by amniocentesis before elective delivery.

Although the ACOG continues to endorse the possibility of a trial of labor after cesarean section in select patients, there are other patients in whom labor is contraindicated [43]. For example, women with a previous classic hysterotomy and women who have previously undergone transfundal uterine surgery or transmural myomectomy are at high risk for uterine rupture [44,45]. Uterine rupture, which can occur in labor or even before the onset of contractions, can be a catastrophic event associated with massive blood loss, significant maternal and fetal morbidity, and maternal and fetal mortality [45,46]. Given the potential for adverse outcomes if labor ensues in women with a prior non–low-transverse hysterotomy, optimal management involves cesarean delivery before the onset of labor. Although many practitioners opt to proceed with delivery at 36 to 37 weeks of gestatio⸱⸱

Box 1. Clinical methods of confirming that a pregnancy has reached 39 completed weeks of gestation

- Fetal heart tones have been documented for 20 weeks by a nonelectronic fetoscope or for 30 weeks by Doppler ultrasonography.
- It has been 36 weeks since a positive serum or urine human gonadotropin pregnancy test was performed by a reliable laboratory.
- An ultrasound measurement of the crown-rump length obtained at 6 to 12 weeks supports a gestational age of at least 39 weeks.
- An ultrasound scan obtained at 13 to 20 weeks confirms the gestational age of at least 39 weeks as determined by clinical history and physical examination.

From American College of Obstetricians and Gynecologists. Induction of labor. Practice bulletin number 10. November 1999; with permission.

---

a gestational age at which the risk for neonatal morbidity is thought to be low and beyond which the risk for labor increases, there remain no clear guidelines regarding the optimal time when cesarean section should be performed in these patients.

Placental disorders: placenta previa, placenta accreta, and placental abruption

Placenta previa is a condition in which the placenta is located in the lower uterine segment and is overlying or immediately adjacent to the internal cervical os. Risk factors for placenta previa include prior uterine surgery (eg, cesarean delivery, dilatation and curettage, hysterotomy), smoking, multifetal gestation, increasing parity, and increasing maternal age [47]. Although many patients who have placenta previa remain stable without antepartum bleeding, vaginal bleeding may occur in response to increased maternal activity, advancing gestation, uterine contractions, and cervical change. The incidence of placenta accreta—defined as an abnormally adherent placenta with trophoblastic tissue invading beyond the decidua to the myometrial surface—has increased significantly as the cesarean section rate has increased and is now a leading cause of postpartum hemorrhage and peripartum hysterectomy [47]. Placental abruption, a condition in which the ˡ⁻⁻⁻ta separates from the uterus prematurely, leading to bleeding that oc- ᵗʰe maternal fetal interface, is becoming more common, with a 23% the rate of abruption noted over the past 2 decades [48]. Risk fac- ᵗtal abruption include maternal hypertension, thrombophilias, tobacco or cocaine use, trauma, and rapid decompression of the uterus [49]. Although abruptions may be asymptomatic or mild and chronic, abruptions may also be acute and lead to rapid maternal or fetal hemorrhage. Any of these placental disorders—previa, accreta, or abruption—may be associated with significant antepartum, intrapartum, and postpartum bleeding, leading to increased morbidity and mortality for the mother and fetus.

In general, expert recommendations call for inpatient observation of women with vaginal bleeding attributable to placenta previa, accreta, or abruption in the second and third trimesters [47,49]. ACSs should be administered to patients between 24 and 34 weeks of gestation at the time of admission [47,49]. Although severe vaginal bleeding accompanied by acute maternal or fetal decompensation is an indication for delivery at any gestational age, supportive care and expectant management are recommended for vaginal bleeding before 34 weeks [47,49]. Beyond 34 weeks, delivery is recommended if labor ensues or vaginal bleeding occurs with the potential for maternal or fetal compromise. Given the increasing risk for hemorrhage associated with advancing gestational age and the risk for increased maternal and fetal morbidity associated with emergent rather than planned delivery, expert opinion supports elective delivery at 36 to 37 weeks of gestation after documentation of fetal lung maturity in those patients who placenta previa or accreta and remain stable to the late preterm period [47]. Guidelines are less clear regarding the recommended management of patients who have a stable chronic abruption, but it seems reasonable to manage these patients similarly with planned delivery at 36 to 37 weeks of gestation after documentation of fetal lung maturity. Unfortunately, existing literature does not offer sufficient data to determine the proportion of late preterm births that result from delivery of patients who have placental disorders, such as previa, accreta, or abruption. Furthermore, US birth records do not document sufficient information to determine whether the late preterm deliveries of patients who have placental disorders occur electively or as a result of appropriate indications.

Maternal medical conditions

Several chronic medical conditions are commonly diagnosed in women of childbearing age. These maternal medical disorders may be associated with adverse pregnancy outcomes or may be exacerbated by pregnancy. Although some women with chronic diseases may go on to have uncomplicated pregnancies with favorable maternal and fetal outcomes, many women experience significant maternal and fetal morbidity during their pregnancy. For example, women with chronic hypertension are at increased risk for intrauterine growth restriction (IUGR), abruption, and PEC [50]. Similarly, systemic lupus erythematosus (SLE) is known to carry with it an increased risk for adverse pregnancy outcome, including an increased risk for preterm delivery, PEC, and fetal loss [51]. Some women with SI ¯

also experience more frequent and severe disease flares during pregnancy [51]. Chronic renal disease is not associated with an increased incidence of adverse pregnancy outcomes, but pregnancy may also lead to permanent worsening of maternal renal function in some women with chronic renal disease. Although poorly controlled pregestational diabetes is associated with an increased risk for miscarriage and fetal structural malformations, pregestational diabetes is also associated with maternal and fetal complications later in gestation.

Volumes of literature have been published on the recommended management of each of these and other medical disorders in pregnancy. In general, physicians caring for women with chronic medical diseases in pregnancy must be vigilant for evidence of maternal or fetal compromise. Close surveillance of maternal and fetal status is indicated with frequent prenatal visits and fetal testing. Worsening of maternal or fetal status in the setting of one of many maternal medical conditions may be cause for delivery, possibly in the preterm or late preterm period. Nevertheless, care must be taken to balance the risks for continuing pregnancy in the setting of maternal or fetal complications against the neonatal risks associated with iatrogenic preterm delivery. Unfortunately, the existing literature does not offer sufficient data to determine the proportion of preterm deliveries among women with coexisting medical conditions that occur electively as opposed to those that occur as a result of appropriate indications.

Fetal indications

Intrauterine growth restriction

IUGR is classically defined as a fetus with an estimated fetal weight decreasing lower than the 10th percentile for the given gestational age [52]. Although many fetuses with estimated weights at less than the 10th percentile are simple constitutionally small fetuses at the lower end of the normal growth spectrum, some fetuses measure lower than the 10th percentile because of suboptimal intrauterine growth. Maternal factors associated with IUGR include coexisting medical disorders (hypertension, chronic renal disease, thrombophilias, hemoglobinopathies, diabetes, and collagen-vascular disorders), malnutrition, tobacco and drug use, and low socioeconomic status [52]. IUGR may also occur in the setting of placental disorders (including abruptions, previa, and hematomas); multiple gestations; or pregnancies complicated by congenital viral infections, aneuploidy, teratogen exposure, and fetal genetic syndromes [52].

Growth-restricted fetuses are at increased risk for antepartum, intrapar-
~~~~ ~nd neonatal complications. Pregnancies complicated by IUGR are at
⅃ risk for oligohydramnios and abnormal intrapartum fetal heart
ʳs and at increased risk for having a cesarean section and low
[52]. Neonatal complications of IUGR include polycythemia,

hyperbilirubinemia, hypoglycemia, and hypothermia in addition to an increased risk for seizures, sepsis, and neonatal death [53]. Management of IUGR remote from term includes close antepartum surveillance, including the use of Doppler ultrasonography to assess umbilical artery waveforms [52].

Recommendations regarding the optimal timing of delivery of a fetus with IUGR are, however, less clear and depend on the gestational age and fetal status. As with any pregnancy, early elective delivery may lead to severe neonatal morbidity and mortality related to prematurity, whereas continued expectant management of an IUGR pregnancy may lead to additional fetal compromise, resulting in acidosis and fetal demise or survival with long-term neurologic sequelae. In preterm pregnancies complicated by IUGR before 34 weeks, expectant management is usually continued unless significantly abnormal testing results develop suggesting fetal compromise. Iatrogenic preterm delivery for IUGR is generally recommended only if testing results are suggestive of fetal acidosis or if abnormal venous Doppler ultrasonography findings are noted [54]. Given the relatively low neonatal mortality associated with delivery beyond 34 weeks, however, delivery is often advocated if IUGR is detected in the setting of hypertension near term [30,54]. Other indications leading to the elective delivery of IUGR fetuses in the late preterm period include lack of fetal growth over serial ultrasound scans, biophysical profile (BPP) with a score of less than 6, or umbilical artery Doppler waveforms with absent or reversed end-diastolic flow at beyond 34 weeks [54]. The optimal timing of delivery has not been determined in the setting of continued reassuring testing, but delivery at term is likely reasonable in most instances. In general, iatrogenic preterm delivery is not indicated for IUGR in the setting of otherwise reassuring fetal testing results.

Oligohydramnios

Oligohydramnios is the term used to describe an amniotic fluid volume that is lower than expected at a given gestational age. The quantitative definition of oligohydramnios, however, varies, with some authorities defining oligohydramnios as no vertical pocket measuring greater than 2 cm [53] and others defining oligohydramnios as an amniotic fluid index of less than 5 [55]. The incidence of oligohydramnios varies based not only on the definition used but on the characteristics and gestational age of the population tested, with oligohydramnios being more common in patients who have maternal medical complications; in patients undergoing indicated ultrasonography for size, date discrepancy, or decreased fetal movement; and in patients at term. The differential diagnosis of oligohydramnios is broad, ranging from fetal structural anomalies to uteroplacental insufficiency or ruptured membranes. Consequences of oligohydramnios occurring in the second trimester include pulmonary hypoplasia and fetal deformations, whereas low amniotic fluid volume predisposes to umbilical cord compression at any gestational age. Although umbilical cord compression is usually transient and results in no long-term consequences, prolonged or repetitive umbilical cord compression may lead to fetal hypoxia and death.

As with so many other conditions, the management of oligohydramnios depends on gestational age, the etiology of the low amniotic fluid volume, and the maternal and fetal status. Because oligohydramnios at term has been associated with an increased risk for meconium staining of the amniotic fluid [56,57], variable decelerations, and an increased risk for cesarean section [58], some consider oligohydramnios at term to be an indication for delivery [58]. The ACOG, however, acknowledges that "an ideal cutoff level for intervention using the AFI has yet to be established" and recommends that management of oligohydramnios be individualized. In the setting of otherwise reassuring fetal testing, the ACOG not only advocates continued expectant management of preterm oligohydramnios but suggests that delivery may be postponed even beyond 37 weeks of gestation [58]. Given the risk associated with low amniotic fluid levels, increased fetal surveillance with nonstress testing and serial assessments of the amniotic fluid volume and fetal growth is recommended in all ongoing pregnancies complicated by oligohydramnios [58].

Despite recommendations for the management of oligohydramnios at term and in preterm pregnancies, the optimal management of oligohydramnios in late preterm period remains unclear. Although there are no specific guidelines calling for elective preterm delivery of patients who have oligohydramnios in the setting of otherwise reassuring fetal testing results, the prospective risk for cord compression and meconium passage may be used to justify delivery in the late preterm period. Data, however, demonstrate that expectant management of oligohydramnios is associated with no increased risk for fetal death [59]. Similarly, multiple additional studies have demonstrated that expectant management of oligohydramnios, even at term, is associated with overall favorable pregnancy outcomes [60–63]. Given the morbidity associated with late preterm delivery, practitioners should be encouraged to manage patients who have uncomplicated oligohydramnios expectantly until term. In accordance with published guidelines, close fetal surveillance should be performed at regular intervals to assess fetal status and delivery should be performed in the setting of nonreassuring fetal testing results [58]. Further research is required to determine the proportion of late preterm deliveries resulting from the delivery of patients who have oligohydramnios, and future efforts should be focused on optimizing fetal testing strategies for oligohydramnios occurring in the late preterm period.

Multiple gestations

Data suggest that the incidence of multiple gestations, including twins and higher order multiples, has increased significantly over the past 2 decades as a result of increasing maternal age attributable to delayed childbearing and the increased use of assisted reproductive technology (ART). By 2005, the number of twin gestations had increased an average of 3% per year since 1980, leading to a 75% increase to an all-time high of 32.2 per 1000 live births [2]. Similarly, the number of triplets, quadruplets, and other higher order births increased more than 400% between 1980 and 1998 [64], with more triplets being delivered in 2003 than in any previous year [41].

Multiple gestations are known to be at increased risk for preterm delivery. The mean gestational age at delivery was 35.3 weeks among twins born in 2002, 32.3 weeks among triplets, and 29.9 weeks among quadruplets [65]. These preterm deliveries occur not only because of a higher incidence of spontaneous PTL and PPROM but because of the increased incidence of PEC, IUGR, and other complications that often necessitate iatrogenic preterm delivery of multiples for maternal or fetal indications [38,66,67]. In addition, multiple gestations face additional unique risks that may increase the risk for preterm delivery. Several studies have described the "prospective risk of fetal death" in ongoing twin pregnancies and have suggested that twin gestations may benefit from delivery before term [66]. The prospective risk for fetal death in a twin pregnancy at 36 to 37 weeks of gestation seems to be equal to the risk for intrauterine fetal demise in a singleton postterm pregnancy [68], whereas the prospective fetal death and twin neonatal mortality intersect at 39 weeks [69]. Lee and colleagues [70], however, noted that monochorionic-diamniotic twins had a higher risk for stillbirth compared with dichorionic-diamniotic twins at each gestational age after 24 weeks, even among "apparently normal" twins with no apparent anomalies or growth abnormalities. In this study, the risk for fetal death in apparently normal monochorionic twin gestations reached a nadir of 2% at 34 weeks [70]. Because data suggest that fetal death cannot be prevented even with close fetal surveillance, elective delivery of monochorionic twin gestations may be justified in the late preterm period [70,71].

Given the high rate of spontaneous preterm delivery associated with multiple pregnancies, significant effort has been focused on attempting to reduce the preterm birth rate among twins and higher order multiples. Although transvaginal cervical length measurement and fetal fibronectin (FFN) collection have been shown to be beneficial in assessing the risk for preterm delivery in multiple gestations, home uterine monitoring has not been proved to offer any improvement in pregnancy outcome [72]. With regard to the prevention of preterm birth, neither bedrest nor prophylactic cervical cerclage has been shown to prevent preterm delivery in multiple gestations [72]. Similarly, multiple studies have shown that use of tocolytics does not improve pregnancy outcomes in multiple gestations, and is, in fact, associated with significantly more increased maternal risk than in singleton pregnancies [72]. Although progesterone supplementation has been shown to decrease the risk for recurrent preterm birth among high-risk women, prophylactic weekly injections of 17-OHP did not lead to decreased rates of preterm birth among twin and triplet gestations [23].

Given the lack of effective treatments to prevent preterm birth among multiples, primary prevention strategies have been developed in an attempt to reduce the overall incidence of multiple gestations. In a joint statement, the ACOG and American Society of Reproductive Medicine recommend limitation of the number of embryos transferred in in vitro fertilization (IVF) cycles in an attempt to reduce the frequency of higher order multiples [73]. Similarly, use of oral and injectable gonadotropic medications should be closely monitored, and insemination cycles with large numbers of mature follicles should be cancelled to limit the number of high-order multiple gestations resulting from ovulation induction. Multifetal pregnancy reduction (MFPR), the process of reducing a multiple gestation to a singleton or twin gestation, has been shown to result in a decreased risk for preterm delivery and improved pregnancy outcome [74,75]. According to the ACOG, women undergoing ART should be counseled extensively regarding the risks associated with such pregnancies, and women diagnosed with higher order multiple gestations should be offered MFPR [76].

Although the ACOG does not endorse an ideal time for the delivery of multiples, the practice bulletin on multiple gestation acknowledges that "fetal and neonatal morbidity and mortality begin to increase in twin and triplet pregnancies extended beyond 37 and 35 weeks, respectively" [72]. In addition, there is a growing body of evidence regarding the risks associated with prospective fetal death in ongoing multiple gestations. Although these data suggest a possible role for elective late preterm delivery to improve perinatal outcomes, the risk for ongoing pregnancy must be balanced against the neonatal risks associated with late preterm delivery. Future research should be focused on understanding the perinatal outcomes of multiples delivered in the late preterm period and on optimizing antenatal fetal testing strategies.

Summary

Although evidence of worsening maternal or fetal status clearly justifies iatrogenic late preterm delivery, many current obstetric practice guidelines routinely suggest delivery between 34 and 37 weeks. Given the increasing rate of late preterm birth and the increased recognition of the morbidity and mortality associated with delivery between 34 and 37 weeks, these standard obstetric practices and practice patterns leading to late preterm birth should be critically evaluated. The possibility of expectant management of some pregnancy complications in the late preterm period should be investigated. Furthermore, prospective research is warranted to investigate the role of ACSs beyond 34 weeks. If ACSs are proved to be beneficial in late preterm and term infants, might there be a role for short-term tocolysis in those patients presenting in spontaneous PTL beyond 34 weeks? Might there be a role for expectant management and ACS administration in those patients who have PPROM beyond 34 weeks? While research is conducted to determine the optimal management strategy of pregnancy complications arising in the late preterm period, physicians and patients need to be counseled regarding the vulnerability of late preterm infants and the potential for iatrogenic prematurity. Hospital guidelines should be developed and enforced to ensure that elective deliveries are not performed before 39 completed weeks of gestation and that fetal lung maturity should be demonstrated when appropriate pregnancy dating cannot be confirmed before elective delivery.

References

[1] Davidoff MJ, Dias T, Damus K, et al. Changes in the gestational age distribution among US singleton births: impact on rates of late preterm birth, 1992 to 2002. Semin Perinatol 2006;30: 8–15.

[2] Martin JA, Hamilton BE, Sutton PD, et al. Births: final data for 2005. Natl Vital Stat Rep 2007;56:1–104.

[3] Escobar GJ, Clark RH, Greene JD. Short-term outcomes of infants born at 35 and 36 weeks gestation: we need to ask more questions. Semin Perinatol 2006;30:28–33.

[4] Clark RH. The epidemiology of respiratory failure in neonates born at an estimated gestational age of 34 weeks or more. J Perinatol 2005;25(4):251–7.

[5] Laptook A, Jackson DL. Cold stress and hypoglycemia in the late preterm ("near-term") infant: impact on nursery of admission. Semin Perinatol 2006;30:77–80.

[6] Neu J. Gastrointestinal maturation and feeding. Semin Perinatol 2006;30:24–7.

[7] Bhutani VK, Johnson L. Kernicterus in late preterm infants cared for as term healthy infants. Semin Perinatol 2006;30:89–97.

[8] Gray RF, Indurkhya A, McCormick MC. Prevalence, stability, and predictors of clinically significant behavior problems in low birth weight children at 3, 5, and 8 years of age. Pediatrics 2004;114:736–43.

[9] Linnet KM, Wisborg K, Agerbo E, et al. Gestational age, birth weight, and the risk of hyperkinetic disorder. Arch Dis Child 2006;91:655–60.

[10] American College of Obstetricians and Gynecologists. Preterm labor. Technical bulletin number 206. June 1995. Available at: http://www.acog.org. Accessed January 2008.

[11] American College of Obstetricians and Gynecologists. Antenatal corticosteroid therapy for fetal maturation. Committee opinion number 27. May 2002. Available at: http://www.acog.org. Accessed January 2008.

[12] NIH State-of-the-Science Conference: cesarean delivery on maternal request. Available at: http://consensus.nih.gov/PREVIOUSSTATEMENTS.htm. Accessed April 9, 2008.

[13] Stutchfield P, Whitaker R, Russell I. Antenatal betamethasone and incidence of neonatal respiratory distress after elective cesarean section: pragmatic randomized trial. Br Med J 2005; 331:662.

[14] Savitz DA, Blackmore CA, Thorp JM. Epidemiologic characteristics of preterm delivery: etiologic heterogeneity. Am J Obstet Gynecol 1991;164:467–71.

[15] Tucker JM, Goldenberg RL, Davis RO, et al. Etiologies of preterm birth in an indigent population: is prevention a logical expectation? Obstet Gynecol 1991;77:343–7.

[16] McIntire DD, Leveno KJ. Neonatal mortality and morbidity rates in late preterm births compared with births at term. Obstet Gynecol 2008;111:35–41.

[17] Goldenberg RL. The management of preterm labor. Obstet Gynecol 2002;100:1020–37.

[18] American College of Obstetricians and Gynecologists. Management of preterm labor. Practice bulletin number 43. May 2003. Available at: http://www.acog.org. Accessed January 2008.

[19] Gyetvai K. Tocolytics for preterm labor: a systematic review. Obstet Gynecol 1999;94: 869–77.

[20] Rebarber A, Cleary Goldman J, Istwan N, et al. Late preterm elective cessation of tocolysis results in an increased incidence of adverse neonatal outcomes in singleton pregnancies. Am J Obstet Gynecol 2007;197:S43.

[21] Meis PJ, Klebanoff M, Thom E, et al. Prevention of recurrent preterm delivery by 17 alpha-hydroxyprogesterone caproate. N Engl J Med 2003;348:2379–85.

[22] Fonseca EB, Bittar RE, Carvalho MH, et al. Prophylactic administration of progesterone by vaginal suppository to reduce the incidence of spontaneous preterm birth in women at increased risk: a randomized placebo-controlled double-blind study. Am J Obstet Gynecol 2003;188:419–24.

[23] Rouse DJ, Caritis SN, Peaceman AM, et al. A trial of 17 alpha-hydroxyprogesterone caproate to prevent prematurity in twins. N Engl J Med 2007;357:454–61.

[24] Fonseca EB, Celik E, Parra M, et al. Progesterone and the risk of preterm birth among women with a short cervix. N Engl J Med 2007;357:462–9.

[25] Mercer BM. Preterm premature rupture of the membranes. Obstet Gynecol 2003;101: 178–93.

[26] American College of Obstetricians and Gynecologists. Preterm premature rupture of membranes. Practice bulletin number 80. April 2007. Available at: http://www.acog.org. Accessed January 2008.

[27] Garite TJ, Keegan KA, Freeman RK, et al. A randomized trial of ritodrine tocolysis versus expectant management in patients with premature rupture of membranes at 25 to 30 weeks of gestation. Am J Obstet Gynecol 1987;157:388–93.

[28] American College of Obstetricians and Gynecologists. Use of progesterone to reduce preterm birth. Committee opinion number 291. November 2003. Available at: http://www.acog.org. Accessed January 2008.

[29] Naef RW 3rd, Allbert JR, Ross EL, et al. Premature rupture of membranes at 34 to 37 weeks' gestation: aggressive versus conservative management. Am J Obstet Gynecol 1998;178: 126–30.

[30] Sibai BM. Diagnosis and management of gestational hypertension and preeclampsia. Obstet Gynecol 2003;102:181–92.

[31] Sibai BM, Caritis SN, Thom E, et al. Prevention of preeclampsia with low-dose aspirin in healthy, nulliparous pregnant women. N Engl J Med 1993;329:1213–8.

[32] Hauth JC, Ewell MG, Levine RJ, et al. Pregnancy outcome in healthy nulliparous women who subsequently developed hypertension. Obstet Gynecol 2000;95:24–8.

[33] Sibai BM, Caritis S, Hauth J, et al. What we have learned about preeclampsia. Semin Perinatol 2003;27:239–46.

[34] Sibai B, Dekker G, Kupferminc M. Pre-eclampsia. Lancet 2005;365:785–99.

[35] American College of Obstetricians and Gynecologists. Diagnosis and management of preeclampsia and eclampsia. Practice Bulletin Number 33. January 2002. Available at: http://www.acog.org. Accessed January 2008.

[36] Sibai BM. Preeclampsia as a cause of preterm and later preterm (near-term) births. Semin Perinatol 2006;30:16–9.

[37] Knuist M, Bonsel GJ, Treffers PE. Intensification of fetal and maternal surveillance in pregnant women with hypertensive disorders. Int J Gynaecol Obstet 1998;61:127–34.

[38] Sibai BM, Caritis S, Hauth J, et al. Hypertensive disorders in twin versus singleton gestations. Am J Obstet Gynecol 2000;182:934–42.

[39] Hnat MD, Sibai BM, Caritis S, et al. Perinatal outcome in women with recurrent preeclampsia compared with women who develop preeclampsia as nulliparas. Am J Obstet Gynecol 2002;186:422–6.

[40] Mendilcioglu I, Trak B, Uner M, et al. Recurrent preeclampsia and perinatal outcome: a study of women with recurrent preeclampsia compared with women with preeclampsia who remained normotensive during their prior pregnancies. Acta Obstet Gynecol Scand 2004;83:1044–8.

[41] Martin JA, Hamilton BE, Sutton PD, et al. Births: final data for 2003. Natl Vital Stat Rep 2005;54(2):1–25.

[42] American College of Obstetricians and Gynecologists. Induction of labor. Practice bulletin number 10. November 1999. Available at: http://www.acog.org. Accessed January 2008.

[43] American College of Obstetricians and Gynecologists. Vaginal birth after previous cesarean delivery. Practice bulletin number 54. July 2004. Available at: http://www.acog.org. Accessed January 2008.

[44] Halperin ME, Moore DC, Hannah WJ. Classical versus low-segment transverse incision for preterm caesarean section: maternal complications and outcome of subsequent pregnancies. Br J Obstet Gynaecol 1988;95:990–6.

[45] Kieser KE, Baskett TF. A 10-year population-based study of uterine rupture. Obstet Gynecol 2002;100:749–53.

[46] Levrant SG, Wingate M. Midtrimester uterine rupture: a case report. J Reprod Med 1996;41: 186–90.

[47] Oyelese Y, Smulian JC. Placenta previa, placenta accreta, and vasa previa. Obstet Gynecol 2006;107:927–41.

[48] Ananth CV, Joseph KS, Demissie K, et al. Trends in twin preterm birth subtypes in the United States, 1989 through 2000: impact on perinatal mortality. Am J Obstet Gynecol 2005;193:1076–82.

[49] Oyelese Y, Ananth CV. Placental abruption. Obstet Gynecol 2006;108:1005–16.

[50] Sibai BM. Chronic hypertension in pregnancy. Obstet Gynecol 2002;100:369–77.

[51] Yasmeen S, Wilkins EE, Field NT, et al. Pregnancy outcomes in women with systemic lupus erythematosus. J Matern Fetal Med 2001;10:91–6.

[52] American College of Obstetricians and Gynecologists. Intrauterine growth restriction. Practice bulletin number 12. January 2000. Available at: http://www.acog.org. Accessed January 2008.

[53] Chamberlain PF, Manning FA, Morrison I, et al. Ultrasound evaluation of amniotic fluid volume: the relationship of marginal and decreased amniotic fluid volumes to perinatal outcome. Am J Obstet Gynecol 1984;150:245–9.

[54] Resnick R. Intrauterine growth restriction. Obstet Gynecol 2002;99:490–6.

[55] Rutherford SE, Phelan JP, Smith CV, et al. The four-quadrant assessment of amniotic fluid volume: an adjunct to antepartum fetal heart rate testing. Obstet Gynecol 1987;70:353–6.

[56] Leveno KJ, Quirk JG Jr, Cunningham FG, et al. Prolonged pregnancy. I. Observations concerning the causes of fetal distress. Am J Obstet Gynecol 1984;150:465–73.

[57] Phelan JP, Platt LD, Yeh SY, et al. The role of ultrasound assessment of amniotic fluid volume in the management of the postdate pregnancy. Am J Obstet Gynecol 1985;151:304–8.

[58] American College of Obstetricians and Gynecologists. Antepartum fetal surveillance. Practice bulletin number 9. November 1999. Available at: http://www.acog.org. Accessed January 2008.

[59] Kreiser D, el-Sayed YY, Sorem KA, et al. Decreased amniotic fluid index in low-risk pregnancy. J Reprod Med 2001;46:743–6.

[60] Zhang J, Troendle J, Meikle S, et al. Isolated oligohydramnios is not associated with adverse perinatal outcomes. BJOG 2004;111:220–5.

[61] Alchalabi HA, Obeidat BR, Jallad MF, et al. Induction of labor and perinatal outcome: the impact of the amniotic fluid index. Eur J Obstet Gynecol Reprod Biol 2006;126:124–7.

[62] Driggers RW, Holcroft CJ, Blakemore KJ, et al. An amniotic fluid index ≤5 cm within 7 days of delivery in the third trimester is not associated with decreasing umbilical arterial pH and base excess. J Perinatol 2004;24:72–6.

[63] Magann EF, Kinsella MJ, Chauhan SP, et al. Does an amniotic fluid index of ≤5 cm necessitate delivery in high-risk pregnancies? A case-control study. Am J Obstet Gynecol 1999; 180:1354–9.

[64] Martin JA, Park MM. Trends in twin and triplet births: 1980–97. Natl Vital Stat Rep 1999; 47:1–16.

[65] Martin JA, Hamilton BE, Sutton PD, et al. Births: final data for 2002. Natl Vital Stat Rep 2003;52:1–113.

[66] Lee YM, Cleary-Goldman J, D'Alton ME. Multiple gestations and late preterm (near-term) deliveries. Semin Perinatol 2006;30:103–12.

[67] Norwitz ER, Edusa V, Park JS. Maternal physiology and complications of multiple preg-
     nancy. Semin Perinatol 2005;29:338–48.
[68] Sairam S, Costeloe K, Thilaganathan B. Prospective risk of stillbirth in multiple-gestation
     pregnancies: a population-based analysis. Obstet Gynecol 2002;100:638–41.
[69] Kahn B, Lumey LH, Zybert PA, et al. Prospective risk of fetal death in singleton, twin, and
     triplet gestations: implications for practice. Obstet Gynecol 2003;102:685–92.
[70] Lee YM, Wylie BJ, Simpson LL, et al. Twin chorionicity and the risk of stillbirth. Obstet Gy-
     necol 2008;111:301–8.
[71] Barigye O, Pasquini L, Galea P, et al. High risk of unexpected late fetal death in monochor-
     ionic twins despite intensive ultrasound surveillance: a cohort study. PLoS Med 2005;2:
     521–7.
[72] American College of Obstetricians and Gynecologists. Multiple gestation: complicated twin,
     triplet, and high-order multifetal pregnancy. Practice bulletin number 56. October 2004.
     Available at: http://www.acog.org. Accessed January 2008.
[73] The Practice Committee of the American Society for Reproductive Technology, the Amer-
     ican Society for Reproductive Medicine. Guidelines on number of embryos transferred. Fer-
     til Steril 2006;86:S51–2.
[74] Evans MI, Ciorica D, Britt DW. Do reduced multiples do better? Best Pract Res Clin Obstet
     Gynaecol 2004;18:601–12.
[75] Evans MI, Berkowitz RL, Wapner RJ, et al. Improvement in outcomes of multifetal preg-
     nancy reduction with increased experience. Am J Obstet Gynecol 2001;184:97–103.
[76] American College of Obstetricians and Gynecologists. Multifetal pregnancy reduction.
     Committee opinion number 369. June 2007. Available at: http://www.acog.org. Accessed
     January 2008.

CLINICS IN
PERINATOLOGY

Clin Perinatol 35 (2008) 361–371

Neonatal Morbidity and Mortality After Elective Cesarean Delivery

Caroline Signore, MD, MPH[a],*,
Mark Klebanoff, MD, MPH[b]

[a]Pregnancy and Perinatology Branch, Eunice Kennedy Shriver National Institute of Child Health and Human Development, National Institutes of Health, Department of Health and Human Services, 6100 Executive Boulevard, Room 4B03, MSC 7510, Bethesda, MD 20892, USA
[b]Division of Epidemiology, Statistics and Prevention Research, Eunice Kennedy Shriver National Institute of Child Health and Human Development, National Institutes of Health, Department of Health and Human Services, 6100 Executive Boulevard, Room 7B03, MSC 7510, Bethesda, MD 20892, USA

The cesarean delivery (CD) rate in the United States reached 30.2% in 2005, an all-time high [1]. Several factors are contributing to this rise: an increase in the rates of first-time, or primary, CD coupled with a decrease in rates of vaginal birth after cesarean (VBAC) are believed major components. In addition to the growing numbers of elective repeat CDs, there is increasing attention to elective cesarean delivery (ECD) without medical or obstetric indications, which may be performed on maternal request. Clinicians and patients considering ECD should undertake a thorough discussion of the risks and benefits of planned ECD versus planned vaginal delivery as related to maternal and infant outcomes.

This article explores the effects of ECD on neonatal morbidity and mortality. Available data are subject to several limitations. There are no randomized trial data comparing outcomes among births from planned ECD versus planned vaginal delivery in otherwise uncomplicated pregnancies; it is possible that such a trial never can be accomplished. Furthermore, it has been difficult to identify and report rates of ECDs in many observational studies because this procedure option may not be included in hospital coding systems or among payers' reimbursable insurance claims. Thus, this

This work was supported in part by the by the Intramural Research Program of the National Institute of Child Health and Human Development.

* Corresponding author.
E-mail address: signorec@mail.NIH.gov (C. Signore).

0095-5108/08/$ - see front matter. Published by Elsevier Inc.
doi:10.1016/j.clp.2008.03.009

article focuses primarily on available data on neonatal outcomes associated with CD without labor, most commonly in the context of elective repeat cesarean and cesarean for breech, recognizing that data from these patient groups may not be fully generalizable to other types of elective CD (eg, CD on maternal request).

Perinatal and infant mortality

For more than 15 years, United States vital statistics data have indicated a 1.5-fold increased risk for neonatal mortality after CD (planned and unplanned) compared with vaginal delivery, although this has been assumed the result of a greater proportion of high-risk pregnancies delivered operatively [2]. Data more specific to ECD in uncomplicated pregnancies are conflicting. In a meta-analysis of nine studies including more than 33,000 women, Mozurkewich and Hutton reported a significant increase in intrapartum and neonatal deaths among term, nonmalformed infants who underwent a trial of labor compared with those who underwent elective repeat CD (odds ratio [OR] 2.05; 95% CI, 1.17–3.57) [3]. A recent United States population-based study of neonatal and infant mortality by mode of delivery among women who had "no indicated risk," however, showed that neonatal mortality was increased more than twofold after birth by cesarean, even after excluding infants who had congenital anomalies and presumed intrapartum hypoxic events (Apgar score <4) and adjusting for demographic and medical covariates [2]. In these studies and others, the reported rates of neonatal death after elective repeat or "no indicated risk" cesareans are low, ranging from 0.01% to 0.17% [2–5].

When considering the risk for neonatal death after ECD, consideration should be given to the competing risk for fetal demise in an ongoing pregnancy. Many investigators have reported an increase in unexplained intrauterine fetal demise rates that begins near term and continues with advancing gestation [6–8]. Smith [9] calculated the cumulative probability of antepartum stillbirth as 0.08% at 38 weeks' gestation rising to 0.34% at 41 weeks' gestation.

In an attempt to reconcile the competing risks for neonatal death after ECD at term and antepartum stillbirth in ongoing term pregnancies, the authors [10] conducted a decision analysis, modeling the probability of perinatal death among a hypothetical cohort of 2,000,000 women who had uncomplicated pregnancies at 39 weeks, half of whom underwent ECD and half managed expectantly. After taking multiple chance probabilities into account, the model estimated that although neonatal deaths were increased among women delivered by elective cesarean, overall perinatal mortality was increased among women managed expectantly, because of the ongoing risk for fetal death in pregnancies that continue beyond 39 weeks. It was estimated that 1441 ECDs need to be performed to prevent one perinatal death (Table 1). In a separate analysis, Hankins and colleagues [7] reached a similar conclusion.

Table 1

Results of decision analyses comparing outcomes among 1 million elective cesarean deliveries and 1 million planned vaginal deliveries: estimated neonatal morbidity and mortality by management strategy

	Elective cesarean delivery at 39 weeks	Expectant management	Number of cesarean deliveries needed to prevent one case[a]
Perinatal deaths	804	1496	1441
Stillbirths	0	1118	
Neonatal deaths	804	378	
Respiratory morbidity (TTN and RDS)	11,000	2524	
Intracranial hemorrhage	490	1007	1934
Brachial plexus injury	410	787	2653
PPH	3700	1488	
Suspected sepsis	20,000	33,211	76
Confirmed sepsis	0	2635	380
Laceration	8000	2464	

Numbers shown are number of cases per million deliveries.

[a] Results shown only for those outcomes estimated to occur more frequently with expectant management.

Adapted from Signore C, Hemachandra A, Klebanoff M. Neonatal mortality and morbidity after elective cesarean delivery versus routine expectant management: a decision analysis. Semin Perinatol 2006;30:288–95; with permission.

Although this type of modeling is subject to limitations [10–13], elective delivery—by cesarean or induction of labor—of a healthy fetus at 39 weeks by accurate dating essentially eliminates the risk for future in utero fetal demise. There are three important caveats. First, the results of these analyses should not be taken as an impetus for elective delivery before 39 weeks. Neonatal deaths increase with each week of decreasing gestational age, such that by 37 weeks, the association between ECD and reduced perinatal mortality seems lost [10], and perinatal deaths may be expected to increase with surgical intervention (Fig. 1). Clinicians should adhere to American College of Obstetricians and Gynecologists (ACOG) practice guidelines for confirming gestational age (or lung maturity) before elective delivery [14].

Second, these analyses assume that a live-born infant whose impending stillbirth was prevented by ECD at 39 weeks has the same risk for neonatal mortality as an infant who would not have died in utero if managed expectantly. This assumption may not hold in reality, as a fetal condition that may predispose to stillbirth at 40 weeks similarly may predispose to neonatal death after a "rescue" delivery at 39 weeks.

Third, calculation of a number needed to treat assumes a causal relationship between exposure—in this case, mode of delivery—and outcome. This assumption also may be contested; existing observational data do not warrant the conclusion that the association between ECD and perinatal death (or other outcomes considered here) is causal. Similarly, it is delivery of an infant that prevents future stillbirth not ECD per se.

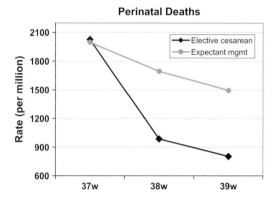

Fig. 1. Estimated perinatal deaths associated with ECD versus expectant management, by gestational age. Perinatal mortality increases for both modes of delivery as gestational age decreases below 39 weeks. At 37 weeks' gestation, more perinatal deaths would be expected with ECD than with expectant management. (*Adapted from* Signore C, Hemachandra A, Klebanoff M. Neonatal mortality and morbidity after elective cesarean delivery versus routine expectant management: a decision analysis. Semin Perinatol 2006;30:288–95; with permission.)

Respiratory morbidity

Although characterized by varying definitions and methodologies, a consistent body of evidence indicates that infants delivered by elective cesarean experience higher rates of respiratory morbidity than infants delivered vaginally [15,16]. In term infants, respiratory difficulty is manifested most often as transient tachypnea of the newborn (TTN), although more serious disorders, such as respiratory distress syndrome (RDS) and persistent pulmonary hypertension (PPH), occur [17,18]. In a cohort study of more than 33,000 births between 37 and 42 weeks, infants delivered by prelabor cesarean (N = 2341) were nearly 7 times more likely to develop respiratory morbidity (RDS or TTN) than infants delivered vaginally (3.6% versus 0.5%; OR 6.8; 95% CI, 5.2–8.9) [19]. In this and other studies [20–22], the risk for respiratory morbidity in term infants is decreased with advancing gestational age. Hansen and colleagues [20] recently showed that infants delivered by elective cesarean at 37 weeks had a 10% incidence of respiratory morbidity (defined as TTN, RDS, or PPH) compared with 2.8% among infants delivered vaginally (OR 3.7; 95% CI, 2.2–6.1). By 40 weeks, the rate of respiratory morbidity with ECD decreased to 1.5% and no longer was significantly different from the rate seen with vaginal deliveries. Even among term infants, respiratory difficulty associated with ECD can be serious. In the Hansen study, 1.9% of infants delivered by ECD at 37 weeks experienced serious respiratory morbidity, defined as that requiring treatment for 3 days or more with continuous oxygen, nasal continuous positive airway pressure, or any period of mechanical ventilation [20].

Proposed mechanisms for the association between CD and respiratory morbidity include iatrogenic prematurity with surfactant deficiency [18,23] and an attenuation of the fetal catecholamine surge during labor [24,25]. Some [19,26], but not all [27,28], investigators report a decrease in respiratory morbidity if CD is performed after onset of labor. This has prompted some investigators to recommend deferral of ECD until after the onset of spontaneous labor [29].

As discussed previously, ACOG practice guidelines specify that without biochemical assessment of fetal lung maturity, elective delivery should not be undertaken before 39 weeks' gestation by strict criteria [14]. This recommendation was affirmed by an expert panel conducting the recent National Institutes of Health and Human Development State-of-the-Science Conference: Cesarean Delivery on Maternal Request [30]. A recent British randomized trial showed that a single course of antenatal corticosteroids before ECD at 37 weeks or later significantly decreased special care nursery admissions for respiratory distress (2.4% versus 5.1%; $P = .021$; relative risk 0.46; 95% CI, 0.23–0.93) [31]. The treatment effect was particularly pronounced at 37 to 38 weeks, but even with treatment, respiratory distress was substantially more common at these gestational ages than at 39 weeks or later. Again, delaying ECD until 39 weeks or later decreases rates of newborn respiratory distress, but steroids may be helpful in preventing respiratory complications in a fetus at 37 or 38 weeks with a nonimmediate indication for prelabor CD.

Neonatal asphyxia or encephalopathy and permanent neurologic injury

Early advocates for ECD proposed that these "atraumatic" deliveries would decrease the risk for intrapartum neurologic injury and cerebral palsy [32]. Neonatal encephalopathy is a clinical syndrome of abnormal neurologic function in late preterm and term infants characterized by altered level of consciousness, abnormal muscular tone and reflexes, respiratory difficulty, or seizure activity [33]. Infants who have neonatal encephalopathy may or may not develop permanent neurologic impairment, such as cerebral palsy. Despite consistently rising CD rates over the past 3 decades, cerebral palsy rates in term (≥ 2500-g) infants have not decreased [34], supporting the widely held premise that a minority of cases (approximately 10%) of encephalopathy and cerebral palsy in these infants are related to intrapartum hypoxic events, thus amenable to prevention by altering route of delivery [35,36]. Alternatively, in at least some cases, ECD at 39 weeks is expected to preempt an unpredictable catastrophic obstetric event (eg, acute placental abruption at 40 weeks) that might result in permanent neurologic injury.

Data addressing the impact of route of delivery on immediate and long-term neurologic outcome are sparse and conflicting. Badawi and colleagues [37] conducted a case-control study of 164 term infants who had moderate to severe newborn encephalopathy and 400 randomly selected control infants and found a lower risk for encephalopathy in infants delivered by elective cesarean (defined as CD planned at least 24 hours before surgery) than in those delivered via spontaneous vaginal delivery (OR 0.17; 95% CI, 0.05–0.56). Alternatively, Towner and colleagues [38] found higher rates of convulsions and central nervous system depression among infants weighing 2500 g to 4000 g delivered by cesarean without labor than in infants delivered spontaneously, although the difference was only significant for central nervous system depression (OR 2.2). A limitation of this study is that the "cesarean without labor" group likely included pregnancies with precarious maternal or fetal status, which would confound the relationship between mode of delivery and neonatal neurologic outcome [16]. Another consideration is that the vaginal delivery comparison groups in both studies consisted of actual spontaneous births, not all births from planned vaginal delivery, some of which would have been vacuum, forceps, and cesarean deliveries during labor. In the Badawi and Towner articles, rates of neonatal neurologic abnormalities were significantly higher in those delivered by operative vaginal delivery (OR 2.3–6.9) and CD during labor (OR 2.2–10.8) compared with spontaneous vaginal delivery [37,38]. If ECD prevents cerebral palsy, given that the United States rate of cerebral palsy is two to three per thousand and that 10% of cases arise intrapartum, approximately 3000 to 5000 ECDs would need to be performed to prevent one case of cerebral palsy related to labor events [10,32,39].

Intracranial hemorrhage

Mode of delivery may be expected to influence rates of intracranial bleeding in neonates (ie, subdural or cerebral, intraventricular, and subarachnoid hemorrhage). Towner and colleagues [38] conducted a large, population-based retrospective review of more than 583,000 births of 2500- to 4000-g infants to nulliparous women in California and found a combined rate of intracranial hemorrhage of 0.4% among operative vaginal deliveries, 0.1% in CDs with labor, 0.05% in spontaneous vaginal deliveries, and 0.05% in CDs without labor. Although risk was significantly increased for operative vaginal delivery and CD during labor, there was no significant difference in the risk for intracranial hemorrhage between women who underwent prelabor CD and those who had a spontaneous vaginal delivery. These data suggest that intracranial hemorrhage may be related to underlying abnormalities of labor, as operative vaginal deliveries and labored CDs often are undertaken because of dysfunctional labor.

Suspected and confirmed neonatal sepsis

Suspected neonatal infection is a major reason for admissions to neonatal intensive care units and invasive procedures in infants. Infection and inflammation are linked to higher rates of cerebral palsy [40,41]. There are scant data comparing rates of suspected and confirmed neonatal sepsis in infants delivered by ECD and by planned vaginal delivery. Hook and colleagues [42] compared infectious outcomes among 497 women undergoing elective repeat CD and 492 who attempted VBAC. Rates of suspected and confirmed neonatal sepsis were significantly lower in the elective repeat CD group (2% versus 5%, $P < .05$ for suspected sepsis, and 0% versus 1% $P < .05$ for proved sepsis). The rate of suspected sepsis was 12% in neonates born after a failed trial of labor compared with 2% after a successful VBAC ($P < .0001$). Based on these data, a decision analytic model estimated that evaluations for suspected neonatal sepsis would be decreased with a policy of ECD at term but that 380 ECDs would need to be performed to prevent one confirmed case of neonatal sepsis [10].

Brachial plexus injury

Shoulder dystocia leading to brachial plexus injury remains a feared complication of attempted vaginal delivery. Shoulder dystocia remains difficult to predict, despite identification of risk factors, such as maternal diabetes, maternal obesity, and fetal macrosomia. Several studies have examined the potential benefit of prophylactic CD for preventing brachial plexus injury to a suspected macrosomic fetus [43–46], but there are few data regarding the impact of ECD on the rate of brachial plexus injury in nonmacrosomic infants. One large population-based study in California examined rates of brachial plexus injuries by mode of delivery in infants weighing 2500 g to 4000 g and found that compared with spontaneous vaginal deliveries, brachial plexus injuries were significantly less common in CDs (0.03% versus 0.08%; OR 0.4; 95% CI, 0.3–0.5) and significantly more common in operative vaginal deliveries (0.5% versus 0.08%; OR 6.0; 95% CI, 3.3–10.7) [38]. Brachial plexus injury occurred in 0.04% of CDs without labor; this rate was not significantly different from that of spontaneous vaginal deliveries (0.08%; OR 0.5; 95% CI, 0.3–1.0) [38].

Fetal lacerations

That infants delivered by cesarean would be at risk for laceration from sharp instruments is intuitive and borne out in published reports. Fetal laceration occurs in 0.1% to 3.1% of CDs [47–52]. The risk for fetal laceration is greater during emergent (5.3%) and unscheduled labored CDs (1.8%) than in ECDs without labor (1.0%) [47,52]. Other risk factors for fetal laceration at CD are abnormal presentation [49,50] and rupture of membranes [52]. Although moderate to severe injuries requiring plastic surgical repair are reported, lacerations that occur during ECD usually are mild and rarely require treatment beyond application of sterile strips [47,52].

Other outcomes

There are limited data examining other outcomes that may be influenced by ECD. Several investigators have expressed concern that CD, by separating mother and infant after birth, may have a negative impact on bonding and early initiation of breastfeeding [53]. In the Term Breech Trial, 77% of women randomized to planned vaginal delivery and 73% randomized to planned CD initiated breastfeeding "within a few hours" of delivery ($P = .05$) [54]. The median duration of breastfeeding was 8 months in both groups [55].

Another area of interest has been the "hygiene hypothesis" (ie, an alteration in microbial colonization of neonates not exposed to vaginal flora during delivery), which may affect postnatal maturation of T cells and predispose to illnesses later in childhood [56]. Several investigators have reported associations between CD and childhood asthma [57–59], but these findings have not been replicated in other studies [60–62].

Summary

Increasing CD rates in the United States and worldwide are of intense interest and public health importance. Elective repeat CD rates have been increasing steadily since the late 1990s, and there may be a growing trend in CDs on maternal request. There are insufficient data on which to base conclusions regarding rates of neonatal morbidity and mortality between planned ECD and planned vaginal delivery. Nevertheless, existing data suggest that ECD is associated with greater risk for neonatal respiratory morbidity and fetal laceration and potentially decreased risk for brachial plexus injury, neonatal sepsis, intracranial hemorrhage, intrapartum asphyxia, and neonatal encephalopathy. Although neonatal deaths may be increased among infants delivered via elective cesarean, overall perinatal mortality may be reduced because of prevention of antepartum stillbirths. To minimize potential neonatal risks in ECDs, these deliveries should not be undertaken before 39 weeks' gestation. Patients considering ECD should be made aware of available data on potential risks and benefits to fetus and neonate. Further research is needed to inform these discussions.

References

[1] Hamilton BE, Martin JA, Ventura SJ. Births: preliminary data for 2005. Natl Vital Stat Rep 2006;55:1–18.
[2] Macdorman MF, Declercq E, Menacker F, et al. Infant and neonatal mortality for primary cesarean and vaginal births to women with "no indicated risk," United States, 1998–2001 birth cohorts. Birth 2006;33:175–82.
[3] Mozurkewich EL, Hutton EK. Elective repeat cesarean delivery versus trial of labor: a meta-analysis of the literature from 1989 to 1999. Am J Obstet Gynecol 2000;183:1187–97.
[4] Richardson BS, Czikk MJ, daSilva O, et al. The impact of labor at term on measures of neonatal outcome. Am J Obstet Gynecol 2005;192:219–26.
[5] Smith GC, Pell JP, Cameron AD, et al. Risk of perinatal death associated with labor after previous cesarean delivery in uncomplicated term pregnancies. JAMA 2002;287:2684–90.

[6] Froen JF, Arnestad M, Frey K, et al. Risk factors for sudden intrauterine unexplained death: epidemiologic characteristics of singleton cases in Oslo, Norway, 1986–1995. Am J Obstet Gynecol 2001;184:694–702.

[7] Hankins GD, Clark SM, Munn MB. Cesarean section on request at 39 weeks: impact on shoulder dystocia, fetal trauma, neonatal encephalopathy, and intrauterine fetal demise. Semin Perinatol 2006;30:276–87.

[8] Yudkin PL, Wood L, Redman CW. Risk of unexplained stillbirth at different gestational ages. Lancet 1987;1:1192–4.

[9] Smith GC. Life-table analysis of the risk of perinatal death at term and post term in singleton pregnancies. Am J Obstet Gynecol 2001;184:489–96.

[10] Signore C, Hemachandra A, Klebanoff M. Neonatal mortality and morbidity after elective cesarean delivery versus routine expectant management: a decision analysis. Semin Perinatol 2006;30:288–95.

[11] Goel V. Decision analysis: applications and limitations. The Health Services Research Group. CMAJ 1992;147:413–7.

[12] Kassirer JP, Moskowitz AJ, Lau J, et al. Decision analysis: a progress report. Ann Intern Med 1987;106:275–91.

[13] Rouse DJ, Owen J. Decision analysis. Clin Obstet Gynecol 1998;41:282–95.

[14] American College of Obstetrics and Gynecology. Induction of labor. ACOG Technical Bulletin [No. 10]. Washington DC: American College of Obstetrics and Gynecology. 1999.

[15] Hansen AK, Wisborg K, Uldbjerg N, et al. Elective caesarean section and respiratory morbidity in the term and near-term neonate. Acta Obstet Gynecol Scand 2007;86:389–94.

[16] Viswanathan M, Visco AG, Hartmann K, et al. Cesarean delivery on maternal request Evidence Report/Technology Assessment No. 133. AHRQ Publication No. 06–E009. Rockville (MD): Agency for Healthcare Research and Quality; 2006.

[17] Keszler M, Carbone MT, Cox C, et al. Severe respiratory failure after elective repeat cesarean delivery: a potentially preventable condition leading to extracorporeal membrane oxygenation. Pediatrics 1992;89:670–2.

[18] Parilla BV, Dooley SL, Jansen RD, et al. Iatrogenic respiratory distress syndrome following elective repeat cesarean delivery. Obstet Gynecol 1993;81:392–5.

[19] Morrison JJ, Rennie JM, Milton PJ. Neonatal respiratory morbidity and mode of delivery at term: influence of timing of elective caesarean section. Br J Obstet Gynaecol 1995;102:101–6.

[20] Hansen AK, Wisborg K, Uldbjerg N, et al. Risk of respiratory morbidity in term infants delivered by elective caesarean section: cohort study. BMJ 2008;336:85–7.

[21] Visco AG, Viswanathan M, Lohr KN, et al. Cesarean delivery on maternal request: maternal and neonatal outcomes. Obstet Gynecol 2006;108:1517–29.

[22] Zanardo V, Simbi AK, Franzoi M, et al. Neonatal respiratory morbidity risk and mode of delivery at term: influence of timing of elective caesarean delivery. Acta Paediatr 2004;93: 643–7.

[23] Wax JR, Herson V, Carignan E, et al. Contribution of elective delivery to severe respiratory distress at term. Am J Perinatol 2002;19:81–6.

[24] Falconer AD, Lake DM. Circumstances influencing umbilical-cord plasma catecholamines at delivery. Br J Obstet Gynaecol 1982;89:44–9.

[25] Faxelius G, Hagnevik K, Lagercrantz H, et al. Catecholamine surge and lung function after delivery. Arch Dis Child 1983;58:262–6.

[26] Gerten KA, Coonrod DV, Bay RC, et al. Cesarean delivery and respiratory distress syndrome: does labor make a difference? Am J Obstet Gynecol 2005;193:1061–4.

[27] Levine EM, Ghai V, Barton JJ, et al. Mode of delivery and risk of respiratory diseases in newborns. Obstet Gynecol 2001;97:439–42.

[28] Sutton L, Sayer GP, Bajuk B, et al. Do very sick neonates born at term have antenatal risks? 2. Infants ventilated primarily for lung disease. Acta Obstet Gynecol Scand 2001;80:917–25.

[29] Cohen M, Carson BS. Respiratory morbidity benefit of awaiting onset of labor after elective cesarean section. Obstet Gynecol 1985;65:818–24.

[30] Anonymous. NIH State-of-the-Science Conference Statement on cesarean delivery on maternal request. NIH Consens State Sci Statements 2006;23:1–29.

[31] Stutchfield P, Whitaker R, Russell I. Antenatal betamethasone and incidence of neonatal respiratory distress after elective caesarean section: pragmatic randomised trial. BMJ 2005; 331:662–4.

[32] Wax JR, Cartin A, Pinette MG, et al. Patient choice cesarean: an evidence-based review. Obstet Gynecol Surv 2004;59:601–16.

[33] American College of Obstetricians and Gynecologists' Task Force on Neonatal Encephalopathy and Cerebral Palsy, American College of Obstetricians and Gynecologists and American Academy of Pediatrics. Neonatal encephalopathy and cerebral palsy: defining the pathogenesis and pathophysiology. Washington, DC: American College of Obstetricians and Gynecologists; 2003.

[34] Paneth N, Hong T, Korzeniewski S. The descriptive epidemiology of cerebral palsy. Clin Perinatol 2006;33:251–67.

[35] Clark SL, Hankins GD. Temporal and demographic trends in cerebral palsy—fact and fiction. Am J Obstet Gynecol 2003;188:628–33.

[36] Scheller JM, Nelson KB. Does cesarean delivery prevent cerebral palsy or other neurologic problems of childhood? Obstet Gynecol 1994;83:624–30.

[37] Badawi N, Kurinczuk JJ, Keogh JM, et al. Intrapartum risk factors for newborn encephalopathy: the Western Australian case-control study. BMJ 1998;317:1554–8.

[38] Towner D, Castro MA, Eby-Wilkens E, et al. Effect of mode of delivery in nulliparous women on neonatal intracranial injury. N Engl J Med 1999;341:1709–14.

[39] Blair E, Stanley FJ. Intrapartum asphyxia: a rare cause of cerebral palsy. J Pediatr 1988;112: 515–9.

[40] Nelson KB, Willoughby RE. Infection, inflammation and the risk of cerebral palsy. Curr Opin Neurol 2000;13:133–9.

[41] Wu YW, Colford JM Jr. Chorioamnionitis as a risk factor for cerebral palsy: a meta-analysis. JAMA 2000;284:1417–24.

[42] Hook B, Kiwi R, Amini SB, et al. Neonatal morbidity after elective repeat cesarean section and trial of labor. Pediatrics 1997;100:348–53.

[43] Boulet SL, Salihu HM, Alexander GR. Mode of delivery and birth outcomes of macrosomic infants. J Obstet Gynaecol 2004;24:622–9.

[44] Herbst MA. Treatment of suspected fetal macrosomia: a cost-effectiveness analysis. Am J Obstet Gynecol 2005;193:1035–9.

[45] Mollberg M, Hagberg H, Bager B, et al. High birthweight and shoulder dystocia: the strongest risk factors for obstetrical brachial plexus palsy in a Swedish population-based study. Acta Obstet Gynecol Scand 2005;84:654–9.

[46] Rouse DJ, Owen J, Goldenberg RL, et al. Determinants of the optimal time in gestation to initiate antenatal fetal testing: a decision-analytic approach. Am J Obstet Gynecol 1995;173: 1357–63.

[47] Haas DM, Ayres AW. Laceration injury at cesarean section. J Matern Fetal Neonatal Med 2002;11:196–8.

[48] Okaro JM, Anya SE. Accidental incision of the fetus at caesarian section. Niger J Med 2004; 13:56–8.

[49] Puza S, Roth N, Macones GA, et al. Does cesarean section decrease the incidence of major birth trauma? J Perinatol 1998;18:9–12.

[50] Smith JF, Hernandez C, Wax JR. Fetal laceration injury at cesarean delivery. Obstet Gynecol 1997;90:344–6.

[51] Wiener JJ, Westwood J. Fetal lacerations at caesarean section. J Obstet Gynaecol 2002;22: 23–4.

[52] Dessole S, Cosmi E, Balata A, et al. Accidental fetal lacerations during cesarean delivery: experience in an Italian level III university hospital. Am J Obstet Gynecol 2004;191: 1673–7.

[53] Rowe-Murray HJ, Fisher JR. Baby friendly hospital practices: cesarean section is a persistent barrier to early initiation of breastfeeding. Birth 2002;29:124–31.

[54] Hannah ME, Hannah WJ, Hodnett ED, et al. Outcomes at 3 months after planned cesarean vs planned vaginal delivery for breech presentation at term: the international randomized Term Breech Trial. JAMA 2002;287:1822–31.

[55] Hannah ME, Whyte H, Hannah WJ, et al. Maternal outcomes at 2 years after planned cesarean section versus planned vaginal birth for breech presentation at term: the international randomized Term Breech Trial. Am J Obstet Gynecol 2004;191:917–27.

[56] Prescott SL, Macaubas C, Smallacombe T, et al. Development of allergen-specific T-cell memory in atopic and normal children. Lancet 1999;353:196–200.

[57] Bager P, Melbye M, Rostgaard K, et al. Mode of delivery and risk of allergic rhinitis and asthma. J Allergy Clin Immunol 2003;111:51–6.

[58] Renz-Polster H, David MR, Buist AS, et al. Caesarean section delivery and the risk of allergic disorders in childhood. Clin Exp Allergy 2005;35:1466–72.

[59] Salam MT, Margolis HG, McConnell R, et al. Mode of delivery is associated with asthma and allergy occurrences in children. Ann Epidemiol 2006;16:341–6.

[60] Juhn YJ, Weaver A, Katusic S, et al. Mode of delivery at birth and development of asthma: a population-based cohort study. J Allergy Clin Immunol 2005;116:510–6.

[61] Maitra A, Sherriff A, Strachan D, et al. Mode of delivery is not associated with asthma or atopy in childhood. Clin Exp Allergy 2004;34:1349–55.

[62] Werner A, Ramlau-Hansen CH, Jeppesen SK, et al. Caesarean delivery and risk of developing asthma in the offspring. Acta Paediatr 2007;96:595–6.

CLINICS IN
PERINATOLOGY

Clin Perinatol 35 (2008) 373–393

Elective Cesarean Section: Its Impact on Neonatal Respiratory Outcome

Ashwin Ramachandrappa, MD, MPH,
Lucky Jain, MD, MBA*

*Department of Pediatrics, Emory University School of Medicine,
2015 Uppergate Drive, Atlanta, GA 30322, USA*

One of the biggest challenges a newborn faces after birth is to make the fast transition from fluid-filled lungs to lungs filled with air. Respiratory morbidity as a result of failure to clear fetal lung fluid is not uncommon, and can be particularly problematic in some infants delivered by elective cesarean section (ECS) without being exposed to labor. The increasing rates of cesarean deliveries in the United States and worldwide have the potential for a significant impact on public health and health care costs because of the morbidity associated with this subgroup. While elective cesarean delivery reduces the occurrence of birth asphyxia, trauma, and meconium aspiration, it increases risk of respiratory distress secondary to transient tachypnea of the newborn (TTN), surfactant deficiency, and pulmonary hypertension. Physiologic events in the last few weeks of pregnancy coupled with the onset of spontaneous labor are accompanied by changes in the hormonal milieu of the fetus and its mother, resulting in preparation of the fetus for neonatal transition. Rapid clearance of fetal lung fluid is a key part of these changes, and is mediated in large part by transepithelial sodium reabsorption through amiloride-sensitive sodium channels in the alveolar epithelial cells, with only a limited contribution from mechanical factors and Starling forces. This article discusses the respiratory morbidity associated with ECS, the physiologic mechanisms underlying fetal lung fluid absorption, and potential strategies for facilitating neonatal transition when infants are delivered by ECS before the onset of spontaneous labor.

* Corresponding author.
E-mail address: ljain@emory.edu (L. Jain).

0095-5108/08/$ - see front matter © 2008 Elsevier Inc. All rights reserved.
doi:10.1016/j.clp.2008.03.006   *perinatology.theclinics.com*

The changing landscape for human deliveries

Cesarean births rose for a 10th straight year in 2006 to a record 31.1% of all deliveries in the United States. This rate is more than 50% higher than in 1996 and is accompanied by a significant drop in the number of women attempting vaginal birth after a previous cesarean delivery (VBAC) (Fig. 1) [1]. Most of the overall increase can be attributed to the increase in the primary cesarean rates from 14.6% in 1996 to 20.3% in 2005. This rise in the primary cesarean rate coupled with the decrease in the VBAC rate (7.9% in 2005) means that women who have a primary cesarean section have a greater than 90% chance of having a repeat cesarean section, further increasing the overall cesarean rate in the future [2]. Among the many reasons cited for this increase are the rising age of women giving birth, a greater number of multiple gestations from fertility treatments, and heightened concerns of physicians and mothers about the risks of vaginal birth. Cesarean births in low-risk or "no-risk" mothers where no medical indication can be identified are on the rise and are often referred to as cesarean delivery at maternal request. Cesarean birth rates are considerably higher in some other parts of the world, especially in Latin America [3–7]. Although indications for the high rate of operative deliveries can vary by region and by maternal choice, up to 35% of these procedures may be performed because the woman has had a previous cesarean delivery [1,8,9].

There have been efforts to reduce this high rate of repeat cesarean sections through attempts at trial of labor (VBAC). In 1980, a consensus development conference on cesarean sections convened by the National Institutes of Health (NIH) concluded that vaginal delivery after a previous low transverse cesarean delivery was a safe and acceptable option [10]. A consensus conference in

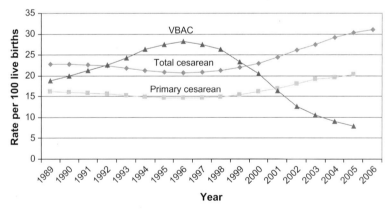

Fig. 1. Rates for total cesarean, primary cesarean, and vaginal birth after cesarean in the United States from 1989 to 2006. For comparability, 2004 and 2005 primary cesarean and VBAC rates are limited to 37 jurisdictions with unrevised birth certificates, encompassing 69% of 2005 births. The total cesarean rate for 2006 is preliminary. (*Data from* U.S. National Center for Health Statistics. Available at: http://www.cdc.gov/nchs/datawh/vitalstats/ VitalStatsbirths.htm. Accessed April 9, 2008.)

Canada in 1985 also arrived at a similar conclusion [11]. The American College of Obstetrics and Gynecology has recommended a trial of labor. Indeed, rates of VBACs rose from 24% in 1980 to 31% in 1991 [8]. However, VBAC rates have fallen by 72% since 1996 [2,12], driven by the fear that trial of labor is associated with more perinatal morbidity and mortality than was previously believed. A large study by McMahon and coworkers [9] showed that major maternal complications (such as uterine rupture) were twice as likely among women who underwent a trial of labor as compared with those who had a second ECS. These investigators suggest that trial of labor is more likely to be successful in a special subset of women, but offer no definitive method for predicting which mothers fall into this group.

Similarly, Smith and coworkers [13], reporting on a population-based study from Scotland that included 313,238 singleton births between 37 and 43 weeks, concluded that, whereas the absolute risk of perinatal death associated with trial of labor following previous cesarean delivery was low, the risk was substantially higher (odds ratio 11.6; 95% CI 1.6–86.7) than that associated with planned repeat cesarean delivery. The investigators also noted a "marked excess of deaths due to uterine rupture compared with other women in labor." Further, 85% of delivery-related perinatal deaths at term among women having a trial of labor occurred at or after 39 weeks' gestation, as did a majority of the antepartum stillbirths (at or after 39 weeks' gestation). A more recent study by Landon and coworkers [14] similarly showed that a trial of labor after prior cesarean delivery is associated with a greater perinatal risk than is elective repeat cesarean delivery without labor, although the absolute risks by any delivery method was low. A further analysis of the same data done by Spong and coworkers [15] confirmed those findings and found increased risks for uterine rupture among women with an indication for cesarean section with labor (0.28%), without labor (0.08%), presence of labor (0.15%), and trial of labor (0.74%), with ECS without labor having the lowest risk (0%). The risk for hypoxic-ischemic encephalopathy was higher in the trial-of-labor group and for those with an indication for cesarean section. Recently Villar and colleagues [16] looked at 97,095 deliveries in a prospective cohort study within the 2005 World Health Organization global survey on maternal and perinatal health and found that among deliveries with cephalic presentation, there was a trend toward a reduced odds ratio for fetal death with ECS (odds ratio 0.65; 95% CI 0.43–0.98) and a larger protective effect with breech presentation. These issues will be covered in greater detail in a forthcoming issue of the Clinics.

Maternal choice: "too posh to push"

Although difficult to quantify, it has been estimated that nearly 4% to 18% of all cesarean deliveries worldwide are done upon maternal request [17]. In the United States, cesarean delivery on maternal request is estimated to be between 2.6% and 5.5% [18]. A recent NIH state-of-the-science consensus seminar, Cesarean Delivery on Maternal Request, reiterates the assertion that maternal request is playing an increasingly important role in obstetricians' decisions to perform cesarean sections [19].

The news media have publicized decisions by such celebrities as Madonna, Britney Spears, Gwyneth Paltrow, and Kate Hudson to choose "elective cesarean" section as their preferred birthing option and have accused them of being "too posh to push" [20,21]. Many obstetricians believe that celebrity pop culture has influenced some women to opt for cesareans without any medical indications. Others, however, believe no credible evidence or study proves this. McCourt and colleagues [21] in their critical review of literature found no evidence of an increasing trend in maternal requests. Surveys by such organizations as Childbirth Connection have found that only 1 in 1600 women planned an ECS, and maternal requests or changing demographics of childbearing women are not the cause of rising cesarean rates [22,23]. Rather, the rising cesarean rates stem from the changing practice standards of medical professionals and their willingness to perform cesarean section because they perceived cesarean deliveries as safer or less likely to lead to malpractice litigation. In fact, nearly one fourth of the mothers surveyed who underwent cesarean section reported pressure from medical personnel to have a cesarean [24].

Most patients and health care providers who prefer cesarean section over vaginal delivery cite as reasons for their preference the greater control and convenience that cesarean section promises and fears associated with vaginal delivery, such as perineal injury, including anal and urinary incontinence, sexual dysfunction, and fetal injury [25]. Because maternal mortality is such a rare occurrence nowadays, evidence showing increased maternal mortality with ECS is insufficient or weak. However, ECS is certainly associated with increased risks for serious maternal morbidity. A British survey of clinicians found that almost half the obstetricians thought that women should be offered their choice of delivery method and 33% of obstetricians in this survey considered a ECS for themselves or their spouses [26]. Their preference for cesarean delivery is due to perceived benefits, such as decreased risk of postpartum hemorrhage, less short-term stress urinary incontinence, lower fetal mortality, reduced probability of hypoxic-ischemic encephalopathy, and lower chances of brachial plexus injury. Table 1 compares the benefits of cesarean delivery with those of vaginal delivery.

Until a reliable method is available that can predict the likelihood of success of trial of labor with minimum morbidity and mortality, or until dramatic changes occur in the cultural, medicolegal, and economic forces, the rate of ECS is likely to stay high and maternal choice is likely to play an increasingly important role.

Respiratory morbidity in infants born by cesarean delivery

Several studies have documented the high incidence of respiratory distress and neonatal intensive care unit (NICU) admissions in infants

Table 1
Comparison of planned vaginal and cesarean section deliveries according to an evidence-based review from Cesarean Delivery on Maternal Request, an NIH state-of-the-science consensus seminar

Evidence quality	Maternal factors	Neonatal factors
Favors planned cesarean section		
Moderate evidence	Less risk of postpartum hemorrhage	
Weak evidence	Less short-term stress urinary incontinence and fewer surgical complications compared with unplanned cesarean deliveries	Less intraventricular hemorrhage, neonatal asphyxia, encephalopathy, brachial plexus injury and neonatal infection
Favors planned vaginal delivery		
Moderate evidence	Reduced length of hospital stay	Less respiratory morbidity
Weak evidence	Lower infection rates; fewer anesthetic complications and thus less subsequent placenta previa; higher breastfeeding rate; lesser risk for uterine rupture and hysterectomy with greater parity	Less iatrogenic prematurity; shorter hospital stays; lower fetal mortality
Neither delivery route offers any advantages	Mortality; anorectal function; sexual function; pelvic organ prolapse; subsequent stillbirth	Mortality; long-term outcomes

Data from Hibbard J, Torre MD. Grand rounds: when mom requests a cesarean. Contemporary OB/GYN 2006:38.

born by cesarean delivery before the onset of spontaneous labor [12,16,21,27–49]. However, the incidence of birth asphyxia, trauma, and meconium aspiration is lower with cesarean delivery, and these advantages of elective cesarean delivery are reviewed in the article by Signore and Klebanoff elsewhere in this issue.

Accurate data about the occurrence of respiratory failure and long-term outcomes in term and near-term infants are hard to obtain because of the lack of large databases, such as those available for preterm infants. However, it is estimated that a significant number of term infants delivered by ECS are admitted to NICUs each year in the United States [50] with the diagnosis of TTN [28,30,36,39,43,49,51–56], respiratory distress syndrome (RDS) [30,36,39,49,53–55], and severe persistent pulmonary hypertension of the newborn/hypoxic respiratory failure [36–38,46]. Some of these reports also show higher rates of mechanical ventilation, oxygen therapy, extracorporeal membrane oxygenation (ECMO), and death. Madar and coworkers

[57] and Roth-Kleiner and coworkers [46] showed that, in infants who develop respiratory distress after ECS, the need for mechanical ventilation was dramatically higher.

Why do elective cesarean deliveries carry a higher risk for the neonate? Because ECS is commonly performed between 37 and 40 weeks' gestation [52], it was believed that at least some of the respiratory morbidity in newborns delivered by ECS was secondary to iatrogenic prematurity [58]. Indeed, studies evaluating large series of patients have shown a higher rate of prematurity [34,59,60] and surfactant deficiency [46,57] in these patients. Several studies have shown that respiratory morbidity in ECS is inversely related to gestational age at the time of ECS [30,36,43]. Hansen and coworkers [36], in a prospective cohort study looking at infants delivered between 37 and 41 weeks' gestation, found that the odds of respiratory morbidity and serious respiratory morbidity were higher among infants at 37, 38, and 39 weeks' gestation delivered by ECS when compared with those delivered vaginally (Fig. 2).

To minimize the occurrence of iatrogenic RDS, fetal lung maturity testing was initially recommended before elective cesarean delivery. However, this is seldom done, given the perception of risks associated with amniocentesis. Also, amniotic fluid testing for fetal lung maturity does not reliably exclude the risk for respiratory distress, as surfactant deficiency is not its sole cause. Changes in the pulmonary vasculature, such as slowing of smooth muscle cell replication and involution at birth, increase in the small pulmonary blood vessels (up to 40 times) in the third trimester, and changes in the epithelial sodium channels with increased ability to clear fetal lung fluid at term and with labor, all play important roles. Delaying ECS to 38 to 40 weeks has been shown to decrease the risk of respiratory distress. However, this carries the risks of spontaneous labor and stillbirths [61]. Further, infants delivered by

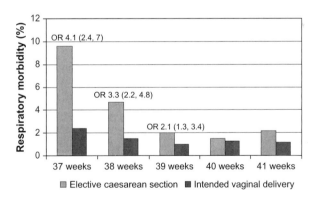

Fig. 2. Neonatal respiratory morbidity after ECS and intended vaginal delivery for 34,458 pregnancies at Aarhus University Hospital, Denmark, 1998–2006. Infants with meconium aspiration syndrome, sepsis, or pneumonia excluded. Adjusted for smoking, alcohol intake, parity, body mass index, marital status, maternal age, and years of schooling. OR, odds ratio. (*Data from* Hansen AK, Wisborg K, Uldbjerg N, et al. Risk of respiratory morbidity in term infants delivered by elective caesarean section: cohort study. BMJ 2008;336:85.)

ECS, in addition to being premature and vulnerable to RDS, are at higher risk for developing TTN (type II RDS, wet lung syndrome) and persistent pulmonary hypertension unrelated to their gestational age at the time of delivery. Although respiratory distress is generally considered to be transient with full recovery and without any long-term consequences, a significant number of infants progress to severe respiratory failure [38]. These infants not only require prolonged hospitalization, but also are at increased risk for chronic lung disease and death [38]. In addition, there is a higher incidence of respiratory depression at birth (low Apgar scores) [53], which is thought to be related to fluid-logged lungs making the transition to air breathing more difficult.

To reduce the occurrence of iatrogenic prematurity associated with ECS deliveries, the American College of Obstetricians and Gynecologists recommends scheduling ECS at 39 weeks or later on the basis of menstrual dates, or waiting for the onset of spontaneous labor. It also lays down the criteria for establishing fetal maturity before ECS [62]. However, as alluded to earlier, the safety of this approach in mothers with previous cesarean section deliveries has not been established in rigorous trials. Some population-based studies [13,15] point to an increased risk of uterine rupture and perinatal death in mothers with previous cesarean section who went into spontaneous labor after 39 weeks. It should also be noted that a vast majority of operative and spontaneous deliveries in the United States occur at community hospitals. Latest data from the Healthcare Cost and Utilization Project shows more deliveries occur in non-teaching hospitals (57%) than teaching hospitals (43%) every year [63]. Data are scant about the accuracy of dating pregnancies at rural hospitals with small delivery services and in pregnancies where prenatal care is initiated late. It is also not clear how rigorously American College of Obstetricians and Gynecologists guidelines for elective cesarean delivery at 39 weeks or later are followed. Such findings, as well as factors related to the convenience of scheduled ECS deliveries for both families and providers, will continue to influence the timing of ECS.

The authors [64] have recently obtained data from the Cesarean Section Registry maintained by the Maternal Fetal Medicine Units Network (MFMU). These data support previously published data on higher occurrence of respiratory distress in infants delivered by elective repeat cesarean section (ERCS) versus those delivered by VBAC. The MFMU Registry tracks infants at or later than 37 weeks' gestation who had an ERCS without any trial of labor, as compared with infants delivered successfully by VBAC. Among infants delivered by ERCS, 6.2% developed respiratory distress and 11.1% required NICU admission, compared with 3.3% respiratory distress and 7.5% NICU admissions in the VBAC group. The registry does not maintain data on the occurrence of pulmonary hypertension of the newborn, ECMO usage, and death, making it difficult to estimate the exact occurrence of hypoxic respiratory failure.

The general impression among clinicians about TTN and "wet lung syndrome" is that of a benign self-limited illness that requires minimal intervention. Although respiratory distress due to TTN and other causes is frequently seen in infants delivered by ECS, it is not clearly known how important this is clinically and how many of these infants become seriously ill and require significant intervention. One approach would be to evaluate the true occurrence of severe hypoxic respiratory failure in this population [65]. Heritage and Cunningham [37] and Keszler and coworkers [38] reported severe respiratory morbidity and resulting mortality in infants born by ECS who developed pulmonary hypertension, giving rise to the term "malignant TTN." A significant number of these infants required ECMO [38]. Previous estimates of ECS-delivered infants in the ECMO population include 16.5% [38], 15% [37], and 17% [66]. The authors recently reviewed data from the ELSO registry to see if this trend had continued since the appearance of reports of ECMO usage in infants delivered by ERCS. From 1986 to 2006, a total of 14,603 infants at or later than 34 weeks' gestation who were treated with ECMO for respiratory failure (excluding diaphragmatic hernia) were analyzed. Infants at or later than 34 weeks and before 37 weeks were labeled "late preterm" and those at or later than 37 weeks were classified as "term." A total of 39.5% of late preterm infants and 37.7% of term infants with hypoxic respiratory failure on ECMO were delivered by ECS (Fig. 3).

The etiology of persistent pulmonary hypertension in newborns delivered by ECS is unclear. Most infants start off as normal or have mild TTN with minimal oxygen requirement and chest radiographs suggestive of retained lung fluid. However, in a subset of infants, there is a gradual increase in oxygen requirement and subsequent evidence of pulmonary hypertension of the newborn. Prematurity is not a significant issue, and these infants do not respond well to surfactant administration [38]. There is considerable

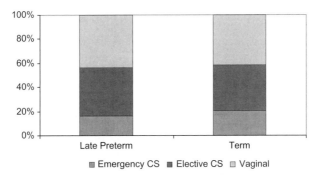

Fig. 3. The mode of delivery of 14,603 infants at or later than 34 weeks who required ECMO in the United States for respiratory failure between 1986 and 2006. Infants with congenital anomalies, such as congenital diaphragmatic hernia, were excluded. Of these infants, 2145 infants were late preterm (defined as at or later than 34 weeks' gestation and before 37 weeks' gestation) and 12,458 term (at or later than 37 weeks' gestation). Infants born by ECS constituted a large fraction of ECMO infants in both subgroups. In contrast, the ECS rate for the study period for the rest of the population was about 10%. CS, cesarean section. (*Data from* The Extracorporeal Life Support Organization registry.)

evidence, especially in the anesthesia literature, that breathing 100% oxygen predisposes patients to atelectasis [67–69]. Looking at adult patients, Rothen and coworkers [69] showed that atelectasis occurs within 5 minutes of breathing 100% oxygen. Benoit and coworkers [67], in a similar study, confirmed these findings. It is common practice to treat mild respiratory distress in term neonates with oxygen hoods or nasal cannula. However, these infants are prone to developing progressive absorption atelectasis, especially when the fraction of inspired oxygen is high. Pulmonary hypertension develops secondarily, and it is not unusual for such infants be in 100% oxygen tents for variable periods of time before they get intubated. A recent Australian study looking at early continuous positive airway pressure versus oxygen hoods found that infants on oxygen hoods requiring high oxygen concentrations were more likely to fail treatment and require a higher level of intensive care than those on continuous positive airway pressure with lower oxygen concentrations [70].

Role of retained fetal lung fluid in neonatal respiratory morbidity

The fetus has an interesting challenge presented to it at birth [64]. Often at short notice, sometimes with no notice at all, it is asked to rapidly clear its air spaces of the fluid that it has been secreting through much of the pregnancy. The ability of a neonate to self-resuscitate at birth after remaining "submerged" in fluid for much of its life is truly remarkable, considering that victims of near-drowning faced with similar amounts of fluid in the lungs do so poorly [64,71,72]. A key player in this process is the lung epithelium, which engineers the switch from placental to pulmonary gas exchange [71,73–80]. For effective gas exchange to occur, alveolar spaces must be cleared of excess fluid and pulmonary blood flow increased to match ventilation with perfusion. Failure of either of these events can jeopardize neonatal transition and cause the infant to develop respiratory distress. We are still far from a complete understanding of the mechanisms by which fetal lungs are able to clear themselves of excessive fluid at birth [81]. It is clear, though, that traditional explanations relying on "Starling forces" and "vaginal squeeze" can only account for a fraction of the fluid absorbed [71,82–86]. Amiloride-sensitive sodium transport by lung epithelia through epithelial sodium channels (ENaC) has emerged as a key event in the transepithelial movement of alveolar fluid [72,74,75,78–80,87–90]. Disruption of this process has been implicated in several disease states, including TTN [91] and hyaline membrane disease [92]. In later life, pulmonary edema can result either from excessive movement of water and solute across the alveolar capillary membrane, or from failure of reabsorption of lung fluid [93,94]. Fig. 4 depicts assembly and regulation of amiloride-sensitive sodium channels in the lung.

Much of what we know about fetal lung fluid dynamics stems from studies of the fetal lamb. Orzaleski and coworkers [95] have shown that, in fetal lambs, lung water content remains fairly constant at 90% to 95%

Epithelial Sodium Channels Diversity:
Mixing and Matching Subunits

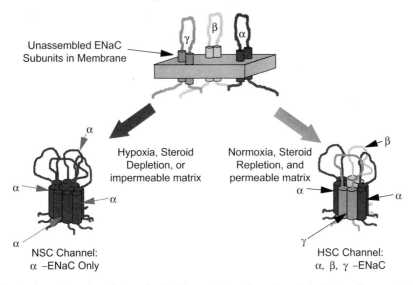

Fig. 4. Assembly and regulation of amiloride-sensitive sodium channels in the lung. Factors in the alveolar environment, particularly oxygen tension, steroid exposure, and alveolar distension, are likely to influence assembly of ENaC subunits. Signal transduction pathways mediated by several protein kinases, including A, G, and C, regulate each of these channel types in different ways. T1 and T2 cells with different channel types (and, therefore, different regulation) have very different levels of sodium transport that respond quite differently to hormonal and transmitter agents. HSC, highly selective cation. NSC, nonselective cation. (*From* Jain L, Eaton DC. Physiology of fetal lung fluid clearance and the effect of labor. Semin Perinatol 2006;30:37; with permission.)

of total lung weight through much of the third trimester. Kitterman and co-workers [96] and others [97,98] found that, in fetal sheep, lung fluid production begins to decrease a few days before spontaneous vaginal delivery and alveolar fluid volume decreases from approximately 25 to 18 mL/kg. Bland and coworkers [73,76,77] showed that preterm delivery and operative delivery without prior labor result in excessive retention of lung fluid in preterm rabbits and in fetal lambs. Sola and Gregory [99] showed that colloid on-cotic pressure varies with mode of delivery and experience of labor, and may influence epithelial fluid absorption. More recently, Berger and coworkers [84] evaluated the effect of lung liquid volume on respiratory performance after cesarean delivery in lamb fetuses. Using chronically catheterized fetal lambs, the investigators found that lambs born with reduced lung liquid volume improved their arterial blood gas and acid base status quicker than those lambs born without a prenatal decrease in their lung liquid volume. This study also confirmed that the experience of vaginal delivery greatly enhances respiratory performance, and this effect is greater than that achieved by simple reduction of lung liquid volume to half in fetuses delivered without enduring labor.

Removal of lung fluid thus started before birth continues postnatally with fluid being carried away by several possible pathways, including pulmonary lymphatics [77,100], blood vessels [101], the upper airway, the mediastinum, and pleural space [102]. There is also recent evidence showing that fetal lung fluid clearance is facilitated by ciliary function [103] and that term neonates with genetic defects of cilia structure or function (primary ciliary dyskinesia) have a high prevalence of neonatal respiratory disease [103].

How is the fetal lung fluid cleared?

It is now clear that active sodium transport across the pulmonary epithelium drives liquid from lung lumen to the interstitium, with subsequent absorption into the vasculature [64,81]. In the lung, sodium reabsorption is a two-step process [104]. The first step is passive movement of sodium from the lumen across the apical membrane into the cell through sodium-permeable ion channels. The second step is active extrusion of sodium from the cell across the basolateral membrane into the serosal space. Several investigators have demonstrated that the initial entry step involves amiloride-sensitive sodium channels. O'Brodovich and coworkers [78], using newborn guinea pigs, have shown that intraluminal instillation of amiloride delays lung fluid clearance. More recent studies using the patch-clamp technique have confirmed the role of alveolar epithelial type I (AT-I) and II (AT-II) cells in the vectorial transport of sodium from the apical surface [87,88,105]. Indeed, complementary DNAs that encode amiloride-sensitive sodium channels in other sodium transporting epithelia have also been cloned from airway epithelial cells [105–107]. The lung epithelium is believed to switch from a predominantly chloride-secreting membrane at birth to a predominantly sodium-absorbing membrane after birth.

Studies in human neonates have also shown that immaturity of sodium transport mechanisms contribute to the development of TTN and RDS [91,92]. Gowen and coworkers [91] were the first to show that human neonates with TTN had an immaturity of the lung epithelial transport, measured as an amiloride-induced drop in potential difference between the nasal epithelium and subcutaneous space. The potential difference was reduced in infants with TTN (suggesting a defect in sodium transport), and recovery from TTN in 1 to 3 days was associated with an increase in potential difference to normal level. Similar studies have now been conducted in premature newborns with hyaline membrane disease, and the results are consistent with impaired sodium transport in these infants [92]. Barker and coworkers [92] measured nasal transepithelial potential difference in 31 premature infants less than 30 weeks' gestation. Nasal potential difference is a good measure of the net electrogenic transport of sodium and chloride (dominant ion) across the epithelial layer (potential difference equals resistance times current), and has been shown to mirror image ion transport occurring in the lower respiratory tract. It is recorded as the potential difference between the mucosal surface of a specific region of the nasal epithelium and the subcutaneous space. Investigators found that maximal nasal epithelial potential difference increased with birthweight and was lower in infants with RDS. Premature infants without RDS had nasal potential difference similar to normal full-term infants. Furthermore, the ability of amiloride to affect the potential difference was lower in preterm infants with RDS on day 1 of life, reflecting lower amiloride-sensitive sodium transport. This study provides important evidence for the role of decreased sodium-channel activity in the pathogenesis of RDS and the accompanying pulmonary edema. There is additional evidence that the ability of various agents to increase lung fluid absorption in fetal lambs is gestational age–dependent [92,97,108–112]. The mechanism for poor response of immature lungs to agents that stimulate sodium transport is not known. Deficiencies could exist in one or more of several steps, including β-receptor, guanosine triphosphate–binding proteins, adenyl cyclase, protein kinase A(PKA), or the sodium channel and its regulatory proteins. Studies have shown that the expression of α-ENaC is developmentally regulated in rats [89] and in humans [110].

Developmental changes in transepithelial ion and fluid movement in the lung can thus be viewed as occurring in three distinct stages [64]. In the first (fetal) stage, the lung epithelium remains in a secretory mode, relying on active chloride secretion via chloride channels and relatively low reabsorption activity of sodium channels. Why the sodium channels remain inactive through much of fetal life is unclear. The second (transitional) stage involves a reversal in the direction of ion and water movement. A multitude of factors may be involved in this transition, including exposure of epithelial cells to an air interface and to high concentrations of steroids and cyclic nucleotides. This stage involves not only increased expression of sodium channels in the lung epithelia, but possibly a switch from nonselective cation channels to highly selective sodium channels. The net increase in sodium movement into the cell can also cause a change in resting membrane potential, leading to a slowing and, eventually, a reversal of the direction of chloride movement through chloride channels. The third and final (adult) stage represents lung epithelia with predominantly sodium reabsorption through sodium channels and possibly chloride reabsorption through chloride channels, with a fine balance between the activity of ion channels and tight junctions. Such an arrangement can help ensure adequate humidification of alveolar surface while preventing excessive buildup of fluid.

What causes the neonatal lung epithelium to switch to an absorptive mode?

Our basic science investigations have focused on physiologic changes that trigger the change in lung epithelia from a chloride-secretory to a sodium-reabsorption mode [64,71,81,87,113,114]. Although several endogenous mediators, including catecholamines, vasopressin, and prolactin, have been proposed to increase lung fluid absorption, none explains this switch convincingly [111,115]. Mechanical factors, such as stretch and exposure of the epithelial cells to air interface, are other probable candidates that have not been well studied. Jain and coworkers [87] have shown that alveolar expression of highly selective sodium channels in the lung epithelia is regulated by the lung microenvironment, especially the presence of glucocorticoids and air interface. Further, regulation of sodium channels is mediated through these factors in a tissue-specific manner [116]. For example, aldosterone is a major factor in the kidney and colon, but probably not in the lung [117]. In the kidneys, it works by activating transcription of genes for ENaC subunits [117]. Of the several factors that have been proposed to have lung-specific effect on sodium reabsorption, some have been investigated, including glucocorticoids, oxygen, β-adrenergics, and surfactant [113,115,118]. Key factors in the lung "microenvironment" are steroids, catecholamines, and oxygen [87,110,119,120]. Based on our animal data and human data from previous studies dealing with preterm gestations, it appears that the most effective strategy for accelerating reabsorption of fetal lung fluid is the administration of exogenous glucocorticoids [121–124].

High doses of glucocorticoids have been shown to stimulate transcription of ENaC in several sodium-transporting epithelia as well as in the lung [110]. In the alveolar epithelia, glucocorticoids were found to induce lung-sodium reabsorption in the late-gestation fetal lung [110]. In addition to increasing transcription of sodium channel subunits, steroids increase the number of available channels by decreasing the rate at which membrane-associated channels are degraded, and increase the activity of existing channels. Glucocorticoids have also been shown to enhance the responsiveness of lungs to β-adrenergic agents and thyroid hormones [125]. The enhanced sodium reabsorption induced by glucocorticoids can be blocked by amiloride, suggesting a role for ENaC. This effect was not observed with triiodothyronine or with cyclic adenosine monophosphate (cAMP). Glucocorticoid induction was found to be receptor-mediated and primarily transcriptional. This observation is important because it provides an alternative explanation for the beneficial effect of antenatal steroids on the lung. This study also confirmed the presence of all three subunits of ENaC in the human fetal lung. O'Brodovich and coworkers [78,89] have shown that, in the rat fetal lung, the expression of α-ENaC is markedly increased at about 20 days' gestation (corresponding to the saccular stage of lung development) and can be accelerated by exposure to dexamethasone and increased levels of thyroid hormone. Such an effect translates into accelerated fetal lung fluid reabsorption at birth. Jain and coworkers [87] have shown that steroids are highly effective in enhancing the expression of highly selective sodium channels in lung epithelial cells. Under conditions of steroid deprivation, alveolar cells express predominantly a nonselective cation channel that is unlikely to transport the large load of sodium and alveolar fluid clearance imposed at birth. However, when these steroid-deprived (both fetal and adult) cells are exposed to dexamethasone, there is rapid transition to highly selective sodium channels, which are readily seen in other sodium- and fluid-transporting systems, such as the kidney and colon [87]. In addition, steroids have been shown to have beneficial effects on the surfactant system as well as pulmonary mechanics [121,124–128].

Can rescue strategies work once an infant has become symptomatic?

Considerable evidence shows that high levels of endogenous catechol-amines at birth may be important for accelerating alveolar fluid clearance [82,85,119]. We [115] have shown that β-agonists increase the activity of sodium channels in the lung through a cAMP-PKA–mediated mechanism. It is logical to conclude that, in the absence of an endogenous surge in fetal catecholamines, exogenous catecholamines should be effective in initiating fetal lung fluid clearance. However, recent studies show that exogenous addition of epinephrine in guinea pigs failed to stimulate fluid clearance in newborn lungs [119]. There are several possible explanations for this finding. First, catecholamines work on the fetal sodium channel (mostly nonselec-tive) by increasing its activity, not by increasing the gene transcription or translation of the proteins required to assemble the channel [64,115]. Thus, if the developmentally regulated ENaC channels are not available in adequate numbers at birth, no amount of extra catecholamines are going to make a difference. Steroids, on the other hand, increase the transcription of the ENaC genes and, through another mechanism involving proteosomal degradation, increase the total number of ENaC channels available at birth. However, a longer duration (4–24 hours) of exposure is required for such an effect. Indeed, if these in vitro findings were to hold true in vivo, then neonates exposed to antenatal steroids would be more responsive to other exogenous agents that enhance sodium channel activity (ie, catecholamines). The authors [129,130] have recently shown that dopamine can greatly enhance sodium channel activity working via a non-cAMP–dependent post-translational mechanism. Because a reduction (~40%) in fetal lung fluid occurs before spontaneous delivery and because rapid clearance of the remaining fluid within hours after birth is essential for successful transition of the fetus, postnatal steroid treatment initiated after the infant has become symptomatic will probably not be a successful alternative strategy.

If cesarean sections are here to stay, can we make them safer?

As mentioned earlier, delaying elective cesarean birth until 39 weeks seems to be the first logical step in reducing iatrogenic prematurity and excess risk of respiratory distress. Risk of respiratory distress and NICU admissions is inversely proportional to the gestational age. Recent analysis of the MFMU network cesarean section registry by Tito and colleagues confirms this. We believe that antenatal glucocorticoids, after having been introduced in 1972 to enhance fetal lung maturity, now have an established role in reducing and preventing life-threatening complications, such as hyaline membrane disease, related to preterm delivery [123,131]. The recommended regimens consist of two 12 mg doses of betamethasone intramuscularly given 12 hours apart or four 6 mg doses of dexamethasone intramuscularly given 4 hours apart [132]. In 1994, an NIH consensus panel strongly recommended the use of antenatal glucocorticoids [132] for preterm pregnancies. In recent years, concern has emerged about the exposure of early gestation preterm fetuses to repeated courses of antenatal steroids [133]. However, a single course has been deemed safe [132]. There has been only one therapeutic trial evaluating the potential use of antenatal betamethasone in term-gestation deliveries by ECS. Stutchfield and coworkers [134] recently reported a randomized pragmatic trial evaluating the efficacy of betamethasone in preventing respiratory distress in infants delivered by ECS. Their results show that two doses of betamethasone given in the 48 hours before delivery significantly decreased admissions due to respiratory distress (5.1% in the control group versus 2.4% in the treatment group; relative risk 0.46, 95% CI 0.23–0.93) (Fig. 5). Similarly, Finer and coworkers [135] have reported their experience with a protocolized approach to congenital diaphragmatic hernia in which congenital diaphragmatic hernia mothers received antenatal dexamethasone at term followed by elective cesarean delivery. Although no control group without these interventions is available for comparison, the investigators

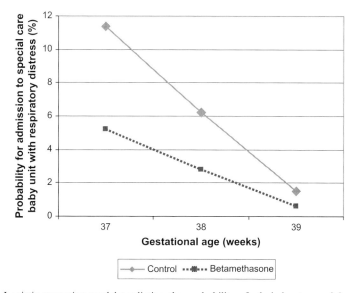

Fig. 5. Logistic regression model predicting the probability of admission to special care baby unit with respiratory distress by gestation, from a randomized trial of 998 mothers scheduled for ECS at term (≥37 weeks). Mothers in the treatment arm (n = 508) received two doses of betamethasone 48 hours before delivery. (*Data from* Stutchfield P, Whitaker R, Russell I. Antenatal betamethasone and incidence of neonatal respiratory distress after elective caesarean section: pragmatic randomized trial. BMJ 2005;331:665.)

reported 78% survival rate. We are currently investigating the safety and efficacy of an antepartum course of betamethasone given for prevention of respiratory morbidity in infants born by ECS.

Summary

In the United States, a significant number of babies each year are delivered by cesarean delivery before onset of spontaneous labor. Although the occurrence of such complications as birth asphyxia, meconium aspiration, and hypoxic-ischemic encephalopathy is reduced, a significant number of these infants develop respiratory distress due to failed transition and may require additional treatments, such as ventilation, surfactant, inhaled nitric oxide, and ECMO. The need is urgent for preventive and therapeutic interventions that can help optimize the outcome of this vulnerable population.

References

[1] Hamilton BE, Martin JA, Ventura SJ. Births: preliminary data for 2006. Natl Vital Stat Rep 2007;56:1–18.
[2] Martin JA, Hamilton BE, Sutton PD, et al. Births: final data for 2005. Natl Vital Stat Rep 2007;56:1–104.
[3] Althabe F, Belizan JM. Caesarean section: the paradox. Lancet 2006;368:1472–3.
[4] Belizan JM, Althabe F, Barros FC, et al. Rates and implications of caesarean sections in Latin America: ecological study. BMJ 1999;319:1397–400.
[5] Belizan JM, Althabe F, Cafferata ML. Health consequences of the increasing caesarean section rates. Epidemiology 2007;18:485–6.
[6] Abitbol MM, Taylor-Randall UB, Barton PT, et al. Effect of modern obstetrics on mothers from third-world countries. J Matern Fetal Med 1997;6:276–80.
[7] Villar J, Valladares E, Wojdyla D, et al. Caesarean delivery rates and pregnancy outcomes: the 2005 WHO global survey on maternal and perinatal health in Latin America. Lancet 2006;367:1819–29.
[8] Centers for Disease Control and Prevention. Rates of cesarean delivery—United States, 1991. MMWR Morb Mortal Wkly Rep 1993;42:285–9.
[9] McMahon MJ, Luther ER, Bowes WA, et al. Comparison of a trial of labor with an elective second cesarean section. N Engl J Med 1996;335:689–95.
[10] US Department of Health and Human Services. Repeat cesarean birth. In: Cesarean Childbirth. Washington, DC: National Institutes of Health; 1981. p. 351–74.
[11] Indications for cesarean section: final statement of the panel of the National Consensus Conference on aspects of cesarean birth. CMAJ 1986;134:1348–52.
[12] Menacker F, Declercq E, Macdorman MF. Cesarean delivery: background, trends, and epidemiology. Semin Perinatol 2006;30:235–41.
[13] Smith GCS, Pell JP, Cameron AD, et al. Risk of perinatal death associated with labor after previous cesarean delivery in uncomplicated term pregnancies. J Am Med Assoc 2002;287:2684–90.
[14] Landon MB, Hauth JC, Leveno KJ, et al. Maternal and perinatal outcomes associated with a trial of labor after prior cesarean delivery. N Engl J Med 2004;351:2581–9.
[15] Spong CY, Landon MB, Gilbert S, et al. Risk of uterine rupture and adverse perinatal outcome at term after cesarean delivery. Obstet Gynecol 2007;110:801–7.
[16] Villar J, Carroli G, Zavaleta N, et al. Maternal and neonatal individual risks and benefits associated with caesarean delivery: multicentre prospective study. BMJ 2007;335:1025.
[17] Wax JR, Cartin A, Pinette MG, et al. Patient choice cesarean: an evidence-based review. Obstet Gynecol Surv 2004;59:601–16.

[18] Declercq E, Menacker F, MacDorman M. Rise in "no indicated risk" primary caesareans in the United States, 1991–2001: cross sectional analysis. BMJ 2005;330:71–2.

[19] National Institutes of Health state-of-the-science conference statement: cesarean delivery on maternal request. Obstet Gynecol 2006;107:1386–97.

[20] Chang L. Elective Cesarean: babies on demand. Available at: http://www.webmd.com/baby/features/elective-cesarean-babies-on-demand. Accessed February 12, 2008.

[21] McCourt C, Weaver J, Statham H, et al. Elective cesarean section and decision making: a critical review of the literature. Birth 2007;34:65–79.

[22] Declercq E, Menacker F, Macdorman M. Maternal risk profiles and the primary cesarean rate in the United States, 1991–2002. Am J Public Health 2006;96:867–72.

[23] Declercq E, Sakala C, Corry M, et al. Listening to mothers II: the second national U.S. survey of women's childbearing experiences. New York: Childbirth Connection; 2006. p. 1.

[24] Why does the national U.S. cesarean section rate keep going up? Available at: http://www.childbirthconnection.org. Accessed February 8, 2008.

[25] Hibbard J, Torre MD. Grand rounds: when mom requests a cesarean. Contemporary ob/gyn 2006;38–50.

[26] Lavender T, Kingdon C, Hart A, et al. Could a randomised trial answer the controversy relating to elective caesarean section? National survey of consultant obstetricians and heads of midwifery. BMJ 2005;331:490–1.

[27] Alderdice F, McCall E, Bailie C, et al. Admission to neonatal intensive care with respiratory morbidity following 'term' elective caesarean section. Ir Med J 2005;98:170–2.

[28] Annibale DJ, Hulsey TC, Wagner CL, et al. Comparative neonatal morbidity of abdominal and vaginal deliveries after uncomplicated pregnancies. Arch Pediatr Adolesc Med 1995; 149:862–7.

[29] Clark RH. The epidemiology of respiratory failure in neonates born at an estimated gestational age of 34 weeks or more. J Perinatol 2005;25:251–7.

[30] Donaldsson SF, Dagbjartsson A, Bergsteinsson H, et al. (Respiratory dysfunction in infants born by elective cesarean section without labor). Laeknabladid 2007;93:675–9 [in Icelandic].

[31] Ersch J, Roth-Kleiner M, Baeckert P, et al. Increasing incidence of respiratory distress in neonates. Acta Paediatr 2007;96:1577–81.

[32] Gerten KA, Coonrod DV, Bay RC, et al. Cesarean delivery and respiratory distress syndrome: does labor make a difference? Am J Obstet Gynecol 2005;193:1061–4.

[33] Gouyon JB, Ribakovsky C, Ferdynus C, et al. Severe respiratory disorders in term neonates. Paediatr Perinat Epidemiol 2008;22:22–30.

[34] Hack M, Fanaroff AA, Klaus MH, et al. Neonatal respiratory distress following elective delivery. A preventable disease? Am J Obstet Gynecol 1976;126:43–7.

[35] Hansen AK, Wisborg K, Uldbjerg N, et al. Elective caesarean section and respiratory morbidity in the term and near-term neonate. Acta Obstet Gynecol Scand 2007;86:389–94.

[36] Hansen AK, Wisborg K, Uldbjerg N, et al. Risk of respiratory morbidity in term infants delivered by elective caesarean section: cohort study. BMJ 2008;336:85–7.

[37] Heritage CK, Cunningham MD. Association of elective repeat cesarean delivery and persistent pulmonary hypertension of the newborn. Am J Obstet Gynecol 1985;152:627–9.

[38] Keszler M, Carbone MT, Cox C, et al. Severe respiratory failure after elective repeat cesarean delivery: a potentially preventable condition leading to extracorporeal membrane oxygenation. Pediatrics 1992;89:670–2.

[39] Kolas T, Saugstad OD, Daltveit AK, et al. Planned cesarean versus planned vaginal delivery at term: comparison of newborn infant outcomes. Am J Obstet Gynecol 2006;195:1538–43.

[40] MacDorman MF, Declercq E, Menacker F, et al. Infant and neonatal mortality for primary cesarean and vaginal births to women with "no indicated risk," United States, 1998–2001 birth cohorts. Birth 2006;33:175–82.

[41] Macdorman MF, Declercq E, Menacker F, et al. Neonatal mortality for low-risk women by method of delivery. Birth 2007;34:101–2.

[42] Many A, Helpman L, Vilnai Y, et al. Neonatal respiratory morbidity after elective cesarean section. J Matern Fetal Neonatal Med 2006;19:75–8.

[43] Morrison JJ, Rennie JM, Milton PJ. Neonatal respiratory morbidity and mode of delivery at term: influence of timing of elective caesarean section. Br J Obstet Gynaecol 1995;102: 101–6.

[44] Parilla BV, Dooley SL, Jansen RD, et al. Iatrogenic respiratory distress syndrome following elective repeat cesarean delivery. Obstet Gynecol 1993;81:392–5.

[45] Ross MG, Beall MH. Cesarean section and transient tachypnea of the newborn. Am J Obstet Gynecol 2006;195:1496–8.

[46] Roth-Kleiner M, Wagner BP, Bachmann D, et al. Respiratory distress syndrome in near-term babies after caesarean section. Swiss Med Wkly 2003;133:283–8.

[47] van den Berg A, van Elburg RM, van Geijn HP, et al. Neonatal respiratory morbidity following elective caesarean section in term infants. A 5-year retrospective study and a review of the literature. Eur J Obstet Gynecol Reprod Biol 2001;98:9–13.

[48] Zanardo V, Padovani E, Pittini C, et al. The influence of timing of elective cesarean section on risk of neonatal pneumothorax. J Pediatr 2007;150:252–5.

[49] Zanardo V, Simbi AK, Franzoi M, et al. Neonatal respiratory morbidity risk and mode of delivery at term: influence of timing of elective caesarean delivery. Acta Paediatr 2004;93: 643–7.

[50] Angus DC, Linde-Zwirble WT, Clermont G, et al. Epidemiology of neonatal respiratory failure in the United States: projections from California and New York. Am J Respir Crit Care Med 2001;164:1154–60.

[51] Fisler RE, Cohen A, Ringer SA, et al. Neonatal outcome after trial of labor compared with elective repeat cesarean section. Birth 2003;30:83–8.

[52] Hales KA, Morgan MA, Thurnau GR. Influence of labor and route of delivery on the frequency of respiratory morbidity in term neonates. Int J Gynaecol Obstet 1993;43:35–40.

[53] Hook B, Kiwi R, Amini SB, et al. Neonatal morbidity after elective repeat cesarean section and trial of labor. Pediatrics 1997;100:348–53.

[54] Levine EM, Ghai V, Barton JJ, et al. Mode of delivery and risk of respiratory diseases in newborns. Obstet Gynecol 2001;97:439–42.

[55] Richardson BS, Czikk MJ, daSilva O, et al. The impact of labor at term on measures of neonatal outcome. Am J Obstet Gynecol 2005;192:219–26.

[56] Riskin A, Abend-Weinger M, Riskin-Mashiah S, et al. Cesarean section, gestational age, and transient tachypnea of the newborn: timing is the key. Am J Perinatol 2005;22: 377–82.

[57] Madar J, Richmond S, Hey E. Surfactant-deficient respiratory distress after elective delivery at 'term'. Acta Paediatr 1999;88:1244–8.

[58] Davidoff MJ, Dias T, Damus K, et al. Changes in the gestational age distribution among U.S. singleton births: impact on rates of late preterm birth, 1992 to 2002. Semin Perinatol 2006;30:8–15.

[59] Goldenberg RL, Nelson K. Iatrogenic respiratory distress syndrome. An analysis of obstetric events preceding delivery of infants who develop respiratory distress syndrome. Am J Obstet Gynecol 1975;123:617–20.

[60] Maisels MJ, Rees R, Marks K, et al. Elective delivery of the term fetus. An obstetrical hazard. J Am Med Assoc 1977;238:2036–9.

[61] Hankins GD, Longo M. The role of stillbirth prevention and late preterm (near-term) births. Semin Perinatol 2006;30:20–3.

[62] American Academy of Pediatrics. American College of Obstetrics and Gynecology: Guidelines for Perinatal Care. 5th edition. American Academy of Pediatrics; 2002. p. 148.

[63] HCUPnet. A tool for identifying, tracking, and analyzing national hospital statistics. Available at: http://hcupnet.ahrq.gov. Accessed April 3, 2008.

[64] Jain L, Eaton DC. Physiology of fetal lung fluid clearance and the effect of labor. Semin Perinatol 2006;30:34–43.

[65] Halliday HL. Elective delivery at "term": implications for the newborn. Acta Paediatr 1999;88:1180–1.

[66] Leder M, Hirschfeld S, Fanaroff A. Persistent fetal circulation: an epidemiologic study. Pediatr Res 1980;14:490.

[67] Benoit Z, Wicky S, Fischer JF, et al. The effect of increased FIO(2) before tracheal extubation on postoperative atelectasis. Anesth Analg 2002;95:1777–81.

[68] Rothen HU, Sporre B, Engberg G, et al. Reexpansion of atelectasis during general anaesthesia may have a prolonged effect. Acta Anaesthesiol Scand 1995;39:118–25.

[69] Rothen HU, Sporre B, Engberg G, et al. Influence of gas composition on recurrence of atelectasis after a reexpansion maneuver during general anesthesia. Anesthesiology 1995; 82:832–42.

[70] Buckmaster AG, Arnolda G, Wright IM, et al. Continuous positive airway pressure therapy for infants with respiratory distress in non tertiary care centers: a randomized, controlled trial. Pediatrics 2007;120:509–18.

[71] Jain L. Alveolar fluid clearance in developing lungs and its role in neonatal transition. Clin Perinatol 1999;26:585–99.

[72] O'Brodovich HM. Respiratory distress syndrome: the importance of effective transport [editorial; comment]. J Pediatr 1997;130:342–4.

[73] Bland RD. Dynamics of pulmonary water before and after birth. Acta Paediatr Scand 1983;(Suppl 305):12–20.

[74] Bland RD. Loss of liquid from the lung lumen in labor: more than a simple "squeeze". Am J Physiol Lung Cell Mol Physiol 2001;280:L602–5.

[75] Bland RD. Lung epithelial ion transport and fluid movement during the perinatal period. Am J Physiol 1990;259:L30–7.

[76] Bland RD, Bressack MA, McMillan DD. Labor decreases the lung water content of newborn rabbits. Am J Obstet Gynecol 1979;135:364–7.

[77] Bland RD, Hansen TN, Haberkern CM, et al. Lung fluid balance in lambs before and after birth. J Appl Physiol 1982;53:992–1004.

[78] O'Brodovich H, Hannam V, Seear M, et al. Amiloride impairs lung water clearance in newborn guinea pigs. J Appl Physiol 1990;68:1758–62.

[79] O'Brodovich HM. Immature epithelial Na+ channel expression is one of the pathogenetic mechanisms leading to human neonatal respiratory distress syndrome. Proc Assoc Am Physicians 1996;108:345–55.

[80] O'Brodovich HM. The role of active Na+ transport by lung epithelium in the clearance of airspace fluid. New Horiz 1995;3:240–7.

[81] Jain L, Eaton DC. Alveolar fluid transport: a changing paradigm. Am J Physiol Lung Cell Mol Physiol 2006;290:L646–8.

[82] Baines DL, Folkesson HG, Norlin A, et al. The influence of mode of delivery, hormonal status and postnatal O2 environment on epithelial sodium channel (ENaC) expression in perinatal guinea-pig lung. J Physiol 2000;522(Pt 1):147–57.

[83] Berger PJ, Kyriakides MA, Smolich JJ, et al. Massive decline in lung liquid before vaginal delivery at term in the fetal lamb. Am J Obstet Gynecol 1998;178:223–7.

[84] Berger PJ, Smolich JJ, Ramsden CA, et al. Effect of lung liquid volume on respiratory performance after caesarean delivery in the lamb. J Physiol 1996;492:905–12.

[85] Berthiaume Y, Broaddus VC, Gropper MA, et al. Alveolar liquid and protein clearance from normal dog lungs. J Appl Physiol 1988;65:585–93.

[86] Berthiaume Y, Staub NC, Matthay MA. Beta-adrenergic agonists increase lung liquid clearance in anesthetized sheep. J Clin Invest 1987;79:335–60.

[87] Jain L, Chen XJ, Ramosevac S, et al. Expression of highly selective sodium channels in alveolar type II cells is determined by culture conditions. Am J Physiol Lung Cell Mol Physiol 2001;280:L646–58.

[88] O'Brodovich H. Epithelial ion transport in the fetal and perinatal lung. Am J Physiol 1991; 261:C555–64.

[89] O'Brodovich H, Canessa C, Ueda J, et al. Expression of the epithelial Na+ channel in the developing rat lung. Am J Physiol 1993;265:C491–6.

[90] O'Brodovich H, Hannam V, Rafii B. Sodium channel but neither Na(+)-H+ nor Na-glucose symport inhibitors slow neonatal lung water clearance. Am J Respir Cell Mol Biol 1991;5:377–84.

[91] Gowen CW Jr, Lawson EE, Gingras J, et al. Electrical potential difference and ion transport across nasal epithelium of term neonates: correlation with mode of delivery, transient tachypnea of the newborn, and respiratory rate. J Pediatr 1988;113:121–7.

[92] Barker PM, Gowen CW, Lawson EE, et al. Decreased sodium ion absorption across nasal epithelium of very premature infants with respiratory distress syndrome. J Pediatr 1997; 130:373–7.

[93] Matthay MA, Berthiaume Y, Staub NC. Long-term clearance of liquid and protein from the lungs of unanesthetized sheep. J Appl Physiol 1985;59:928–34.

[94] Matthay MA, Landolt CC, Staub NC. Differential liquid and protein clearance from the alveoli of anesthetized sheep. J Appl Physiol 1982;53:96–104.

[95] Orzalesi MM, Motoyama EK, Jacobson HN, et al. The development of the lung of lambs. Pediatrics 1965;35:373–81.

[96] Kitterman JA, Ballard PL, Clements JA, et al. Tracheal fluid in fetal lambs: spontaneous decrease prior to birth. J Appl Physiol 1979;47:985–9.

[97] Brown MJ, Olver RE, Ramsden CA, et al. Effects of adrenaline and of spontaneous labour on the secretion and absorption of lung liquid in the fetal lamb. J Physiol 1983;344:137–52.

[98] Dickson KA, Maloney JE, Berger PJ. Decline in lung liquid volume before labor in fetal lambs. J Appl Physiol 1986;61:2266–72.

[99] Sola A, Gregory GA. Colloid osmotic pressure of normal newborns and premature infants. Crit Care Med 1981;9:568–72.

[100] Humphreys PW, Normand IC, Reynolds EO, et al. Pulmonary lymph flow and the uptake of liquid from the lungs of lamb at the start of breathing. J Physiol 1967;193:1–29.

[101] Raj JU, Bland RD. Lung luminal liquid clearance in newborn lambs. Effect of pulmonary microvascular pressure elevation. Am Rev Respir Dis 1986;134:305–10.

[102] Cummings JJ, Carlton DP, Poulain FR, et al. Lung luminal liquid is not removed via the pleural space in health newborn lambs. Physiologist 1989;32:202.

[103] Noone PG, Leigh MW, Sannuti A, et al. Primary ciliary dyskinesia: diagnostic and phenotypic features. Am J Respir Crit Care Med 2004;169:459–67.

[104] Matthay MA, Folkesson HG, Verkman AS. Salt and water transport across alveolar and distal airway epithelia in the adult lung. Am J Physiol 1996;270:L487–503.

[105] Voilley N, Lingueglia E, Champigny G, et al. The lung amiloride-sensitive Na+ channel: biophysical properties, pharmacology, ontogenesis, and molecular cloning. Proc Natl Acad Sci U S A 1994;91:247–51.

[106] Canessa CM, Horisberger JD, Rossier BC. Epithelial sodium channel related to proteins involved in neurodegeneration [see comments]. Nature 1993;361:467–70.

[107] Canessa CM, Schild L, Buell G, et al. Amiloride-sensitive epithelial Na+ channel is made of three homologous subunits. Nature 1994;367:463–7.

[108] Barker PM, Brown MJ, Ramsden CA, et al. The effect of thyroidectomy in the fetal sheep on lung liquid reabsorption induced by adrenaline or cyclic AMP. J Physiol 1988; 407:373–83.

[109] Perks AM, Cassin S. The effects of arginine vasopressin and epinephrine on lung liquid production in fetal goats. Can J Physiol Pharmacol 1989;67:491–8.

[110] Venkatesh VC, Katzberg HD. Glucocorticoid regulation of epithelial sodium channel genes in human fetal lung. Am J Physiol 1997;273:L227–33.

[111] Wallace MJ, Hooper SB, Harding R. Regulation of lung liquid secretion by arginine vasopressin in fetal sheep. Am J Physiol 1990;258:R104–11.

[112] Walters DV, Ramsden CA, Olver RE. Dibutyryl cAMP induces a gestation-dependent absorption of fetal lung liquid. J Appl Physiol 1990;68:2054.

[113] Jain L, Chen XJ, Brown LA, et al. Nitric oxide inhibits lung sodium transport through a cGMP-mediated inhibition of epithelial cation channels. Am J Physiol 1998;274:L475–84.

[114] Jain L, Chen XJ, Malik B, et al. Antisense oligonucleotides against the alpha-subunit of ENaC decrease lung epithelial cation-channel activity. Am J Physiol 1999;276:L1046–51.

[115] Chen XJ, Eaton DC, Jain L. Beta-adrenergic regulation of amiloride-sensitive lung sodium channels. Am J Physiol Lung Cell Mol Physiol 2002;282:L609–20.

[116] Renard S, Voilley N, Bassilana F, et al. Localization and regulation by steroids of the alpha, beta and gamma subunits of the amiloride-sensitive Na+ channel in colon, lung and kidney. Pflugers Arch 1995;430:299–307.

[117] Eaton D, Ohara A, Ling BN. Cellular regulation of amiloride blockable Na$^+$ channels. Biomed Res 1991;12:31–5.

[118] Guidot DM, Modelska K, Lois M, et al. Ethanol ingestion via glutathione depletion impairs alveolar epithelial barrier function in rats. Am J Physiol Lung Cell Mol Physiol 2000;279:L127–35.

[119] Finley N, Norlin A, Baines DL, et al. Alveolar epithelial fluid clearance is mediated by endogenous catecholamines at birth in guinea pigs. J Clin Invest 1998;101:972–81.

[120] Mustafa SB, DiGeronimo RJ, Petershack JA, et al. Postnatal glucocorticoids induce alpha-ENaC formation and regulate glucocorticoid receptors in the preterm rabbit lung. Am J Physiol Lung Cell Mol Physiol 2004;286:L73–80.

[121] Ervin MG, Berry LM, Ikegami M, et al. Single dose fetal betamethasone administration stabilizes postnatal glomerular filtration rate and alters endocrine function in premature lambs. Pediatr Res 1996;40:645–51.

[122] Goldenberg RL, Jobe AH. Prospects for research in reproductive health and birth outcomes. J Am Med Assoc 2001;285:633–9.

[123] Liggins GC, Howie RN. A controlled trial of antepartum glucocorticoid treatment for prevention of the respiratory distress syndrome in premature infants. Pediatrics 1972;50:515–25.

[124] Pillow JJ, Hall GL, Willet KE, et al. Effects of gestation and antenatal steroid on airway and tissue mechanics in newborn lambs. Am J Respir Crit Care Med 2001;163:1158–63.

[125] Jobe AH, Ikegami M, Padbury J, et al. Combined effects of fetal beta agonist stimulation and glucocorticoids on lung function of preterm lambs. Biol Neonate 1997;72:305–13.

[126] Smith LM, Ervin MG, Wada N, et al. Antenatal glucocorticoids alter postnatal preterm lamb renal and cardiovascular responses to intravascular volume expansion. Pediatr Res 2000;47:622–7.

[127] Willet KE, Jobe AH, Ikegami M, et al. Lung morphometry after repetitive antenatal glucocorticoid treatment in preterm sheep. Am J Respir Crit Care Med 2001;163:1437.

[128] Willet KE, Jobe AH, Ikegami M, et al. Antenatal endotoxin and glucocorticoid effects on lung morphometry in preterm lambs. Pediatr Res 2000;48:782–8.

[129] Helms MN, Chen XJ, Ramosevac S, et al. Dopamine regulation of amiloride-sensitive sodium channels in lung cells. Am J Physiol Lung Cell Mol Physiol 2006;290:L710–22.

[130] Helms MN, Self J, Bao HF, et al. Dopamine activates amiloride-sensitive sodium channels in alveolar type I cells in lung slice preparations. Am J Physiol Lung Cell Mol Physiol 2006;291:L610–8.

[131] Crowley PA. Antenatal corticosteroid therapy: a meta-analysis of the randomized trials, 1972 to 1994. Am J Obstet Gynecol 1995;173:322–35.

[132] NIH Consensus Development Panel on the Effect of Corticosteroids for Fetal Maturation on Perinatal Outcomes. Effect of corticosteroids for fetal maturation on perinatal outcomes. J Am Med Assoc 1995;273:413–8.

[133] Jobe AH. Glucocorticoids in perinatal medicine: misguided rockets? J Pediatr 2000;137:1–3.

[134] Stutchfield P, Whitaker R, Russell I. Antenatal betamethasone and incidence of neonatal respiratory distress after elective caesarean section: pragmatic randomised trial. BMJ 2005;331:662.

[135] Finer NN, Tierney A, Etches PC, et al. Congenital diaphragmatic hernia: developing a protocolized approach. J Pediatr Surg 1998;33:1331–7.

ELSEVIER
SAUNDERS

CLINICS IN
PERINATOLOGY

Clin Perinatol 35 (2008) 395–406

Cesarean Delivery and Its Impact on the Anomalous Infant

Shannon E.G. Hamrick, MD

*Department of Pediatrics, Emory University, Emory Children's Center,
2015 Uppergate Drive, Atlanta, GA 30322, USA*

A cesarean delivery frequently is performed for anomalous fetal conditions on the grounds that it reduces the risk for birth trauma (from dystocia or to the exposed tissue) and risk for infection to a surgical site. Available data do not always support a fetal benefit from this delivery management, however. Clear evidence of benefit from cesarean delivery is not available for most conditions, and the rarity of individual lesions has prevented randomized controlled trials to assess delivery modes and outcomes. Thus, most studies are retrospective in design or contain very small patient numbers. Furthermore, significant bias exists in many of these studies: typically patients in the cesarean delivery groups were diagnosed prenatally and may have benefited from anticipatory planning, whereas patients in the vaginal delivery group often were born undiagnosed and had to be transported before definitive treatment. To the contrary, prenatal diagnosis may be a marker for a more severe defect; thus, the expected outcomes would be worse. Confounding in either direction makes the interpretation of existing data difficult.

The risks of cesarean delivery to mothers and newborns are well described; they include anesthetic risks, maternal infection, risk for subsequent placenta previa or uterine rupture, longer maternal and neonatal hospital stay, iatrogenic prematurity, and difficulties with transition, including transient tachypnea of newborns or respiratory distress syndrome (RDS) necessitating neonatal intensive care [1]. Benefits of a planned cesarean delivery also are characterized, although by weaker-quality evidence. Lower rates of stress incontinence, lower rates of surgical complications for planned (versus unplanned) cesarean deliveries, fewer birth injuries or lacerations, and reduced neonatal asphyxia, intracranial hemorrhages, and newborn infections have been recognized [1]. A more detailed discussion of the pros and

E-mail address: shannon_hamrick@oz.ped.emory.edu

0095-5108/08/$ - see front matter © 2008 Elsevier Inc. All rights reserved.
doi:10.1016/j.clp.2008.03.005   *perinatology.theclinics.com*

cons of cesarean delivery in general can be found elsewhere in this issue in the articles by Signore and Klebanoff; Ramachandrappa and Jain; and Sharma and Spearman; the focus of this article is the additional considerations that may have an impact on delivery of anomalous infants.

Much of the existing literature on cesarean delivery for anomalous infants describes a primary outcome that is "neonatal mortality" (morbidity unspecified) or an outcome pertinent to the congenital defect (eg, motor function with myelomeningocele). It is rare to be shown data on RDS or other potentially iatrogenic neonatal conditions due to delivery mode, although many of these would be confounded by the postoperative clinical course. Information about the impact of such elective deliveries on mothers also is limited, making it difficult to assess the net risk/benefit to the mother-infant unit; availability of such information would be invaluable in counseling patients. The goal of this review is to summarize the literature on mode of delivery for a variety of fetal diagnoses, describing, where possible, the effect on neonatal morbidities.

Neural tube defects

Neural tube defects (NTD) result from a failure of fusion of the embryologic neural folds. Severe NTD include very high myelomeningocele, myelomeningocele with severe hydrocephalus, anencephaly, and occipital encephalocele with affected neural tissue. In cases where fetal outcome is expected to be dismal, risk to the pregnant woman should be minimized, including not offering a cesarean delivery for fetal indications.

Myelomeningocele

The appropriate delivery mode for myelomeningocele has been controversial for decades. An autopsy study comparing vaginal breech to vaginal vertex delivery revealed increased nerve trauma in the breech fetuses that had NTD; thus, cesarean delivery was advocated for breech presentation [2]. It then was suggested that abdominal delivery might avoid unnecessary trauma to exposed neural tissue and reduce infection to an operative site in all cases [3]. A series of retrospective studies ensued that compared vaginal and abdominal modes of delivery (Table 1) [4–11]. To summarize, no study that looked at short-term outcomes (including meningitis, ventriculoperitoneal shunt placement, and hospital stay) showed a difference in short-term outcomes. In four of the six studies that looked at long-term neurologic outcome, no differences were found [4,7,9,10]. One study showed a benefit in ambulatory status after cesarean delivery for breech presentations, although the vaginal breech-delivered patients eventually had function comparable to the cesarean delivery patients, and the vaginal vertex deliveries had a higher proportion of independent ambulation than elective cesarean deliveries [5].

Table 1
Comparison of retrospective studies evaluating outcomes for myelomeningocele after cesarean or vaginal delivery

First author	Year	Patient numbers vaginal delivery/cesarean delivery	Outcome
Bensen	1988	40/32	No difference in survival, meningitis, or neurologic outcomes at 12 months
			19 Pre-labor CS, 13 with labor CS
Sakala	1990	20/15	No difference in outcomes, including meningitis or ventriculoperitoneal shunt placement
Cochrane	1991	137/71	No difference in ambulatory status
			34 Pre-labor CS, 37 with labor CS. Of VD, 14 were vaginal breech deliveries
Luthy	1991	78/82	Pre-labor CS showed improved motor function at 2 years; significant differences existed between groups with respect to anatomic level
			47 Pre-labor CS, 35 with labor CS
Hill	1994	15/10 (pre-labor)	No difference in short-term motor outcomes
Merrill	1998	22/17	No difference in long-term motor outcomes
Lewis	2004	43/44 (pre-labor)	Trial of labor group showed improved ambulatory status at 2 and 10 years although no difference when controlled for anatomic level
			Trial of labor; 10 of 43 had CS
Preis	2005	29/25	No difference in mortality or ambulatory status; overall mortality rate was 40%

Abbreviations: CS, cesarean delivery; VD, vaginal delivery.

In the largest study that looked at long-term outcome, there was an improvement in motor outcome in the pre-labor cesarean group compared with delivery after the onset of labor [8]. This study suffered from some of the aforementioned biases, however: the planned cesarean patients were diagnosed and followed prenatally. Additionally, there were significant differences between groups for gestational age at delivery, interval between delivery and surgical correction, and anatomic meningomyelocele level.

It has been suggested that a sac size of greater than 6 cm should be delivered by cesarean to prevent sac disruption [11,12] although it is unclear if sac disruption is of clinical significance or might occur in any mode of delivery [7]. Similarly, it has been suggested that a breech presentation (typically higher lesions, above L4) should be delivered operatively [2,5]. Recovery has been noted after perinatal trauma to the neural placode, and there is no guarantee that cesarean delivery is less traumatic [5].

As a whole, this body of literature reports insufficient data for potentially iatrogenic neonatal conditions, so comorbidities, such as RDS or hypoglycemia, are unknown.

Thus, there are no definitive data to support improved short- or long-term outcomes from cesarean delivery for myelomeningocele. The most likely determinant of long-term outcome is anatomic level and associated anomalies (severe hydrocephalus) rather than mode of delivery.

Hydrocephalus (isolated)

The most common cause of isolated hydrocephalus is aqueductal stenosis, although the cause and presence of associated anomalies (including karyotypic) strongly affect prognosis [13]. The prenatal distinction between maximal hydrocephalus and hydranencephaly is difficult to make but critically important with respect for outcome potential [14,15]. Advances in fetal MRI have led to improvements in accurate antenatal diagnosis of central nervous system abnormalities [16,17]. Fetal hydrocephalus with macrocephaly and associated anomalies indicating a dismal prognosis can be offered cephalocentesis and vaginal delivery. Fetuses with ventriculomegaly but no macrocephaly can be offered vaginal delivery. An examination of the literature reveals only case series or other retrospective reviews; these suggest that fetal hydrocephalus with macrocephaly (biparietal diameter greater than 10 cm at term) should be delivered abdominally to reduce the risk for dystocia [12,18–20]. A recent nationwide survey from Japan noted that in 89 patients who had fetal hydrocephalus and 12-month clinical outcome data available, although the majority (76%) were delivered by cesarean, there was a trend toward better neurodevelopmental outcome after vaginal delivery (not statistically significant and biparietal diameter not given) [21]. In each of these reports, data are not given on neonatal respiratory comorbidities.

Cystic hygroma

Cystic hygroma is a malformation of lymphatic vessels and frequently (up to 60%) is seen in conjunction with other abnormalities, including chromosomal abnormalities. When associated with aneuploidy or fetal hydrops, the prognosis is dismal; delivery management should minimize risk to the pregnant woman. There are no data showing a fetal benefit due to mode of delivery. Large anterior lesions, however, may occlude the airway; thus, a planned operative cesarean followed by fetal bronchoscopy, resection if indicated, and endotracheal intubation should be considered (ie, ex utero intrapartum treatment [EXIT] procedure) [22–24].

Sacrococcygeal teratoma

Sacrococcygeal teratomas present a prenatal management and delivery problem when they are large or when they are particularly vascular with resultant high output failure and fetal hydrops and risk for tumor hemorrhage. In these cases, an atraumatic abdominal delivery is warranted. One small experience of 10 cases recommends attempted vaginal delivery if a tumor is less than 5 cm [25]. Fetal surgery is recommended when hydrops develops in the early third trimester [26]. Prompt delivery is indicated if fetal hydrops is causing maternal illness (the mirror syndrome).

Anterior abdominal wall defects

The optimal mode of delivery for anterior abdominal wall defects, including gastroschisis and omphalocele, has been debated extensively in the literature [12,19,27–51]. As with myelomeningoceles, these data are retrospective and limited by selection bias (ie, the antenatally diagnosed and followed inborn patient delivered by cesarean) plus confounded by the inclusion of laboring patients in the cesarean group.

Gastroschisis

Gastroschisis, a paraumbilical wall deformation, most likely is the result of a vascular accident that disrupts normal abdominal wall development. Although it is associated less frequently with chromosomal anomalies than omphalocele, it is associated with other intestinal abnormalities, such as atresias and malrotation [52,53]. The past 2.5 decades have produced at least 16 retrospective studies designed to evaluate outcome of gastroschisis based on mode of delivery (Table 2) [27,29,30,32,33,35,36,38–43,46–48]. Recognizing the bias inherent in these retrospective studies, a summary follows. Ten studies detected no difference in "outcome" between cesarean and vaginal deliveries [27,29,32,33,36,39,43,46–48]. Outcome was defined

Table 2

Comparison of retrospective studies designed to evaluate outcomes for gastroschisis after cesarean or vaginal delivery

First author	Year	Patient numbers vaginal delivery/ cesarean delivery	Outcome
Kirk	1983	65/9	No difference in newborn survival or morbidity
Lenke	1986	17/7	Lower mortality and shorter hospital stay with CS
Bethel	1989	14/14	No difference in newborn survival or morbidity
Moretti	1990	41/15	No difference in newborn survival or morbidity
Sipes	1990	23/9	No difference in newborn survival or hospital stay
Lewis	1990	20/29	No difference in newborn survival or morbidity; data pooled for gastroschisis and omphalocele
Sakala	1993	12/15	Less sepsis and shorter hospital stay for CS
Adra	1996	26/16	No difference in newborn survival or morbidity
Quirk	1996	25/31	Longer hospital stay for CS
Snyder	1999	115/68	No difference in newborn survival or morbidity
Dunn	1999	29/31	Staged repair more frequent with VD
How	2000	32/38	No difference in newborn survival or morbidity
Malas	2002	18/22	No survival difference; shorter hospital stay for CS
Singh	2003	102/79	No difference in mortality, ventilation days, infections, hospital stay
Salihu	2004	174/180	No survival difference
Puligandla	2004	82/31	No survival difference; CS associated with increased respiratory distress

Abbreviations: CS, cesarean delivery; VD, vaginal delivery.

differently: neonatal survival; morbidity, such as short bowel syndrome; length of stay; sepsis; duration of total parenteral nutrition; and so forth. Six studies detected a difference in outcome between delivery mode, four favoring cesarean [30,35,38,42], predominantly for length of hospital stay, and two favoring vaginal delivery [40,41]. Most studies did not delineate respiratory distress as a separate outcome; one study showed an incidence of 16.1% in the cesarean group versus 3.7% in the vaginal delivery group ($P = .035$) [40]. Most studies did not differentiate between patients who had and did not have labor in the cesarean groups, a potentially important confounder. A meta-analysis of 15 observational studies determined that there is no relationship between mode of delivery and ability to undergo primary repair and no relationship to newborn sepsis or other newborn morbidity or length of stay [44]. Thus, the consensus suggests no benefit to cesarean delivery, but only a randomized prospective trial will allow for a satisfactory resolution to this debate.

Omphalocele

Omphalocele, an abdominal wall defect characterized by an amnioperitoneal membrane covering herniated intra-abdominal contents, is believed to result from a malformation as opposed to a deformation, such as gastroschisis. It represents a persistence of the primitive stalk with failure of the bowel to return to the abdomen and failure to complete lateral body wall closure. The diagnoses often is complicated by the presence of other visceral (50%–70%) and chromosomal abnormalities (7%–50%) [37,54,55]. Prognosis is more closely dependent on associated anomalies and gestational age at delivery rather than mode of delivery [37,56]. Although definitive data are lacking, cesarean delivery is recommended for cases of extracorporeal liver and cases of "giant" omphalocele (> 5 cm) [37]. Similar to gastroschisis, the available data suggest no benefit for cesarean delivery except as noted for extracorporeal liver and giant omphalocele [33,36,37,39,45,47].

Congenital diaphragmatic hernia

Even with antenatal diagnosis and management, congenital diaphragmatic hernia (CDH) is associated with a high mortality and significant morbidity [57]. Developing a protocolized approach to care, although not necessarily with respect to delivery mode, improves outcomes [58–60]. Ideally, infants who have CDH should be delivered in a center that has neonatal intensive care, pediatric surgery, and availability of extracorporeal membrane oxygenation (ECMO) support, if parents desire comprehensive efforts. Hypothetic benefits from either mode of delivery can be argued: the physiologic impact on pulmonary function and longer gestational time from spontaneous labor versus the optimal timing of an elective delivery for the many resources required [61]. Retrospective data from the Congenital Diaphragmatic Hernia Study Group on 1039 term or near-term infants who had CDH were collected to evaluate if mode of delivery was associated with differences in survival [61]. The overall survival was not different between patients delivered by elective cesarean (71%), induced vaginal delivery (70%), or spontaneous vaginal delivery (67%) [61]. At 30 days of age, survival on room air also was not different between groups: elective cesarean (45%), induced vaginal delivery (37%), or spontaneous vaginal delivery (37%) [61]. Statistically significant survival without use of ECMO was higher in the elective cesarean group, however [61]. Morbidity was not assessed in this study. Prospective studies designed to evaluate mode of delivery and outcomes for CDH are needed, but interpreting these data will be difficult given the heterogeneity of disease.

Skeletal dysplasias

Skeletal dysplasias, such as nonlethal osteogenesis imperfecta (OI), represent a challenging delivery scenario because the mother also may be affected, influencing mode of delivery. Old maternal fractures from OI may result in cephalopelvic disproportion necessitating a cesarean delivery. An attempt at vaginal delivery is recommended except in cases of maternal pelvic fracture or evidence of fetal fractures. Collagen abnormalities associated with OI, however, put the mother at risk for uterine atony and rupture [19,62,63].

Hydrops

Fetal hydrops results from a variety of causes in addition to the aforementioned masses, including congenital heart disease or arrhythmias, twin-twin transfusion, chromosomal abnormalities, hematologic abnormalities (immune and nonimmune anemia), congenital viral infections, and congenital chylothorax [64]. Unless a lethal cause is identified and no intervention is done on behalf of the fetus, cesarean deliveries avoid abdominal dystocia and reduce trauma to edematous and friable fetal tissues.

Hydronephrosis

Abdominal dystocia resulting from hydronephrosis or other fetal genitourinary abnormalities (persistent urogenital sinus with hydrocolpos or fetal ovarian cysts) is rare and there are no data to support cesarean over vaginal delivery for these cases [65–67].

Cardiac anomalies

In general, fetuses with structural congenital heart lesions are not affected by mode of delivery. Fetuses with complete congenital heart block, however, cannot be assessed for tolerance of labor using standard measures. Complete congenital heart block is associated most commonly with atrial isomerism (heterotaxy syndromes) or maternal autoimmune disease [68]. In the absence of hydrops, the use of ultrasound and fetal scalp blood sampling is advocated to achieve a safe vaginal delivery [68–70].

Conjoined twins

Conjoined twinning, a variant of monozygotic twinning, occurs from an abnormal cleavage event on days 13 to 15 post fertilization [71]. A high incidence of dystocia and risk for cord entanglement suggests the need for cesarean delivery after documentation of fetal lung maturity [68,71].

Other

There are several extremely rare lesions with exposed viscera (eg, encephalocele, bladder exstrophy, and cardiac exstrophy) in which cesarean delivery often is performed in cases of antenatal diagnosis [72–74]. Supportive data are lacking but the incidence of such conditions precludes prospective studies.

Summary

The available data do not suggest a benefit for cesarean delivery for most anomalous infants, although the decision must be made individually. The literature on cesarean delivery for anomalous infants reports insufficient information on comorbid neonatal conditions, so these complications are unknown in this population of newborns. In a minority of cases, cesarean delivery is reasonable to prevent dystocia or optimize outcome, including hydrocephalus with macrocephaly; anterior cystic hygroma without associated anomalies; large, vascular sacrococcygeal teratomas; giant omphalocele or omphalocele with extracorporeal liver; nonlethal OI with fetal or maternal fractures; and nonlethal hydrops fetalis. Areas for future investigation include prospective, randomized controlled trials of pre-labor cesarean compared with vaginal delivery for myelomeningocele and anterior abdominal wall defects. The relative rarity of other lesions likely precludes a randomized controlled trial.

References

[1] NIH. NIH state-of-the-science conference statement on cesarean delivery on maternal request. NIH Consens State Sci Statements 2006;23:1–29.
[2] Ralis ZA. Traumatizing effect of breech delivery on infants with spina bifida. J Pediatr 1975; 87:613–6.
[3] Chervenak FA, Duncan C, Ment LR, et al. Perinatal management of meningomyelocele. Obstet Gynecol 1984;63:376–80.
[4] Bensen JT, Dillard RG, Burton BK. Open spina bifida: does cesarean section delivery improve prognosis? Obstet Gynecol 1988;71:532–4.
[5] Cochrane D, Aronyk K, Sawatzky B, et al. The effects of labor and delivery on spinal cord function and ambulation in patients with meningomyelocele. Childs Nerv Syst 1991;7:312–5.
[6] Hill AE, Beattie F. Does caesarean section delivery improve neurological outcome in open spina bifida? Eur J Pediatr Surg 1994;4(Suppl 1):32–4.
[7] Lewis D, Tolosa JE, Kaufmann M, et al. Elective cesarean delivery and long-term motor function or ambulation status in infants with meningomyelocele. Obstet Gynecol 2004; 103:469–73.
[8] Luthy DA, Wardinsky T, Shurtleff DB, et al. Cesarean section before the onset of labor and subsequent motor function in infants with meningomyelocele diagnosed antenatally. N Engl J Med 1991;324:662–6.
[9] Merrill DC, Goodwin P, Burson JM, et al. The optimal route of delivery for fetal meningomyelocele. Am J Obstet Gynecol 1998;179:235–40.

[10] Preis K, Swiatkowska-Freund M, Janczewska I. Spina bifida—a follow-up study of neonates born from 1991 to 2001. J Perinat Med 2005;33:353–6.

[11] Sakala EP, Andree I. Optimal route of delivery for meningomyelocele. Obstet Gynecol Surv 1990;45:209–12.

[12] Anteby EY, Yagel S. Route of delivery of fetuses with structural anomalies. Eur J Obstet Gynecol Reprod Biol 2003;106:5–9.

[13] Volpe JJ. Neurology of the newborn. 4th edition. Philadelphia: W.B. Saunders; 2001.

[14] McAbee G, Chan A, Erde EL. Prolonged survival with hydranencephaly: report of two patients and literature review. Pediatr Neurol 2000;23:80–4.

[15] Sutton LN, Bruce DA, Schut L. Hydranencephaly versus maximal hydrocephalus: an important clinical distinction. Neurosurgery 1980;6:34–8.

[16] Blaicher W, Prayer D, Mittermayer C, et al. The clinical impact of magnetic resonance imaging in fetuses with central nervous system anomalies on ultrasound scan. Ultraschall Med 2005;26:29–35.

[17] Glenn O, Barkovich J. Magnetic resonance imaging of the fetal brain and spine: an increasingly important tool in prenatal diagnosis: part 2. AJNR Am J Neuroradiol. 2006;27:1807–14.

[18] Chervenak FA, Berkowitz RL, Tortora M, et al. The management of fetal hydrocephalus. Am J Obstet Gynecol 1985;151:933–42.

[19] Kuller JA, Katz VL, Wells SR, et al. Cesarean delivery for fetal malformations. Obstet Gynecol Surv 1996;51:371–5.

[20] Pretorius DH, Davis K, Manco-Johnson ML, et al. Clinical course of fetal hydrocephalus: 40 cases. AJR Am J Roentgenol 1985;144:827–31.

[21] Moritakea K, Nagaia H, Nagasakoa N, et al. Diagnosis of congenital hydrocephalus and delivery of its patients in Japan. Brain Dev, in press.

[22] Hirose S, Farmer DL, Lee H, et al. The ex utero intrapartum treatment procedure: looking back at the EXIT. J Pediatr Surg 2004;39:375–80.

[23] Kathary N, Bulas DI, Newman KD, et al. MRI imaging of fetal neck masses with airway compromise: utility in delivery planning. Pediatr Radiol 2001;31:727–31.

[24] Mychaliska GB, Bealer JF, Graf JL, et al. Operating on placental support: the ex utero intrapartum treatment procedure. J Pediatr Surg 1997;32:227–30.

[25] Gross SJ, Benzie RJ, Sermer M, et al. Sacrococcygeal teratoma: prenatal diagnosis and management. Am J Obstet Gynecol 1987;156:393–6.

[26] Harrison MR. Fetal surgery. Am J Obstet Gynecol 1996;174:1255–64.

[27] Adra AM, Landy HJ, Nahmias J, et al. The fetus with gastroschisis: impact of route of delivery and prenatal ultrasonography. Am J Obstet Gynecol 1996;174:540–6.

[28] Axt R, Quijano F, Boos R, et al. Omphalocele and gastroschisis: prenatal diagnosis and peripartal management. A case analysis of the years 1989–1997 at the Department of Obstetrics and Gynecology, University of Homburg/Saar. Eur J Obstet Gynecol Reprod Biol 1999;87: 47–54.

[29] Bethel CA, Seashore JH, Touloukian RJ. Cesarean section does not improve outcome in gastroschisis. J Pediatr Surg 1989;24:1–3.

[30] Dunn JC, Fonkalsrud EW, Atkinson JB. The influence of gestational age and mode of delivery on infants with gastroschisis. J Pediatr Surg 1999;34:1393–5.

[31] Fitzsimmons J, Nyberg DA, Cyr DR, et al. Perinatal management of gastroschisis. Obstet Gynecol 1988;71:910–3.

[32] How HY, Harris BJ, Pietrantoni M, et al. Is vaginal delivery preferable to elective cesarean delivery in fetuses with a known ventral wall defect? Am J Obstet Gynecol 2000;182:1527–34.

[33] Kirk EP, Wah RM. Obstetric management of the fetus with omphalocele or gastroschisis: a review and report of one hundred twelve cases. Am J Obstet Gynecol 1983;146:512–8.

[34] Lenke R. Modern obstetric management and outcome of infants with gastroschisis. Obstet Gynecol 1999;94:638–9.

[35] Lenke RR, Hatch EI Jr. Fetal gastroschisis: a preliminary report advocating the use of cesarean section. Obstet Gynecol 1986;67:395–8.

[36] Lewis DF, Towers CV, Garite TJ, et al. Fetal gastroschisis and omphalocele: is cesarean section the best mode of delivery? Am J Obstet Gynecol 1990;163:773–5.

[37] Lurie S, Sherman D, Bukovsky I. Omphalocele delivery enigma: the best mode of delivery still remains dubious. Eur J Obstet Gynecol Reprod Biol 1999;82:19–22.

[38] Malas NO, Al-Ghoweri AS, Shwyiat RM. The outcome and analysis of 40 cases of fetal gastroschisis. Saudi Med J 2002;23:1083–6.

[39] Moretti M, Khoury A, Rodriquez J, et al. The effect of mode of delivery on the perinatal outcome in fetuses with abdominal wall defects. Am J Obstet Gynecol 1990;163: 833–8.

[40] Puligandla PS, Janvier A, Flageole H, et al. Routine cesarean delivery does not improve the outcome of infants with gastroschisis. J Pediatr Surg 2004;39:742–5.

[41] Quirk JG Jr, Fortney J, Collins HB 2nd, et al. Outcomes of newborns with gastroschisis: the effects of mode of delivery, site of delivery, and interval from birth to surgery. Am J Obstet Gynecol 1996;174:1134–8.

[42] Sakala EP, Erhard LN, White JJ. Elective cesarean section improves outcomes of neonates with gastroschisis. Am J Obstet Gynecol 1993;169:1050–3.

[43] Salihu HM, Emusu D, Aliyu ZY, et al. Mode of delivery and neonatal survival of infants with isolated gastroschisis. Obstet Gynecol 2004;104:678–83.

[44] Segel SY, Marder SJ, Parry S, et al. Fetal abdominal wall defects and mode of delivery: a systematic review. Obstet Gynecol 2001;98:867–73.

[45] Sermer M, Benzie RJ, Pitson L, et al. Prenatal diagnosis and management of congenital defects of the anterior abdominal wall. Am J Obstet Gynecol 1987;156:308–12.

[46] Singh SJ, Fraser A, Leditschke JF, et al. Gastroschisis: determinants of neonatal outcome. Pediatr Surg Int 2003;19:260–5.

[47] Sipes SL, Weiner CP, Sipes DR 2nd, et al. Gastroschisis and omphalocele: does either antenatal diagnosis or route of delivery make a difference in perinatal outcome? Obstet Gynecol 1990;76:195–9.

[48] Snyder CL. Outcome analysis for gastroschisis. J Pediatr Surg 1999;34:1253–6.

[49] Snyder CL, St Peter SD. Trends in mode of delivery for gastroschisis infants. Am J Perinatol 2005;22:391–6.

[50] Strauss RA, Balu R, Kuller JA, et al. Gastroschisis: the effect of labor and ruptured membranes on neonatal outcome. Am J Obstet Gynecol 2003;189:1672–8.

[51] Vegunta RK, Wallace LJ, Leonardi MR, et al. Perinatal management of gastroschisis: analysis of a newly established clinical pathway. J Pediatr Surg 2005;40:528–34.

[52] Novotny DA, Klein RL, Boeckman CR. Gastroschisis: an 18-year review. J Pediatr Surg 1993;28:650–2.

[53] Snyder CL, Miller KA, Sharp RJ, et al. Management of intestinal atresia in patients with gastroschisis. J Pediatr Surg 2001;36:1542–5.

[54] Gilbert WM, Nicolaides KH. Fetal omphalocele: associated malformations and chromosomal defects. Obstet Gynecol 1987;70:633–5.

[55] Yazbeck S, Ndoye M, Khan AH. Omphalocele: a 25-year experience. J Pediatr Surg 1986;21: 761–3.

[56] Nakayama DK, Harrison MR, Gross BH, et al. Management of the fetus with an abdominal wall defect. J Pediatr Surg 1984;19:408–13.

[57] Harrison MR, Adzick NS, Estes JM, et al. A prospective study of the outcome for fetuses with diaphragmatic hernia. JAMA 1994;271:382–4.

[58] Downard CD, Jaksic T, Garza JJ, et al. Analysis of an improved survival rate for congenital diaphragmatic hernia. J Pediatr Surg 2003;38:729–32.

[59] Finer NN, Tierney A, Etches PC, et al. Congenital diaphragmatic hernia: developing a protocolized approach. J Pediatr Surg 1998;33:1331–7.

[60] Harrison MR, Keller RL, Hawgood SB, et al. A randomized trial of fetal endoscopic tracheal occlusion for severe fetal congenital diaphragmatic hernia. N Engl J Med 2003;349: 1916–24.

[61] Frenckner BP, Lally PA, Hintz SR, et al. Prenatal diagnosis of congenital diaphragmatic hernia: how should the babies be delivered? J Pediatr Surg 2007;42:1533–8.

[62] Carlson JW, Harlass FE. Management of osteogenesis imperfecta in pregnancy. A case report. J Reprod Med 1993;38:228–32.

[63] Sharma A, George L, Erskin K. Osteogenesis imperfecta in pregnancy: two case reports and review of literature. Obstet Gynecol Surv 2001;56:563–6.

[64] Abrams ME, Meredith KS, Kinnard P, et al. Hydrops fetalis: a retrospective review of cases reported to a large national database and identification of risk factors associated with death. Pediatrics 2007;120:84–9.

[65] Geifman-Holtzman O, Crane SS, Winderl L, et al. Persistent urogenital sinus: prenatal diagnosis and pregnancy complications. Am J Obstet Gynecol 1997;176:709–11.

[66] Kurjak A, Latin V, Mandruzzato G, et al. Ultrasound diagnosis and perinatal management of fetal genito-urinary abnormalities. J Perinat Med 1984;12:291–312.

[67] Sakala EP, Leon ZA, Rouse GA. Management of antenatally diagnosed fetal ovarian cysts. Obstet Gynecol Surv 1991;46:407–14.

[68] McCurdy CM Jr, Seeds JW. Route of delivery of infants with congenital anomalies. Clin Perinatol 1993;20:81–106.

[69] Schmidt KG, Ulmer HE, Silverman NH, et al. Perinatal outcome of fetal complete atrioventricular block: a multicenter experience. J Am Coll Cardiol 1991;17:1360–6.

[70] Sherman SJ, Featherstone LS. Congenital complete heart block and successful vaginal delivery. J Perinatol 1997;17:489–91.

[71] Graham GM 3rd, Gaddipati S. Diagnosis and management of obstetrical complications unique to multiple gestations. Semin Perinatol 2005;29:282–95.

[72] Chervenak FA, Isaacson G, Mahoney MJ, et al. Diagnosis and management of fetal cephalocele. Obstet Gynecol 1984;64:86–91.

[73] Grethel EJ, Hornberger LK, Farmer DL. Prenatal and postnatal management of a patient with pentalogy of cantrell and left ventricular aneurysm. A case report and literature review. Fetal Diagn Ther 2007;22:269–73.

[74] Kaya H, Oral B, Dittrich R, et al. Prenatal diagnosis of cloacal exstrophy before rupture of the cloacal membrane. Arch Gynecol Obstet 2000;263:142–4.

ELSEVIER
SAUNDERS

Clin Perinatol 35 (2008) 407–420

The Impact of Cesarean Delivery on Transmission of Infectious Agents to the Neonate

Dolly Sharma, MD, Paul Spearman, MD*

Pediatric Infectious Diseases, Emory University School of Medicine, 2015 Uppergate Drive, Atlanta, GA 30322, USA

The rate of cesarean deliveries has dramatically increased over the past decade, with approximately 30% of neonates delivered by this method [1,2]. Statistics have shown that indications for this major procedure have also changed over time, with increasing rates of cesarean sections performed in low-risk women [3]. Cesarean delivery on maternal request has been a hotly debated topic; 40% to 54% of physicians approve of a woman's right to request a cesarean section in the absence of a medical indication [4]. Research to date has not been conclusive in establishing whether the impetus for medically elective cesarean deliveries originates from the providing physician or from maternal request. Studies have highlighted several factors that contribute to the choice of cesarean delivery. Maternal reasons include fear of childbirth, fear of pain, perineal injury, convenience, safer delivery, stress or anxiety, and fear of vaginal examination, whereas physician reasons include patient's fear of childbirth, patient pain, perineal injury, fetal injury, fear of incontinence, patient and physician convenience, and fear of litigation [1]. Interestingly, infection was not cited as an indication for cesarean delivery by obstetricians or their patients in this study. There are relatively few indications for performing cesarean delivery to avoid transmission of infectious agents to the neonate, and the existing indications are unlikely to contribute substantially to the increase in cesarean deliveries. In this review, the authors outline those infections known to be transmitted intrapartum through the infected birth canal and highlight the recommendations for cesarean section attributable to maternal infections.

This article was supported in part by training support for D. Sharma provided by Children's Healthcare of Atlanta.

* Corresponding author.

E-mail address: paul.spearman@emory.edu (P. Spearman).

Herpes simplex virus

Herpes simplex viruses (HSVs) are large double-stranded DNA viruses that commonly infect human populations worldwide. HSV-1 is commonly acquired during childhood through oral mucosal exposure to infected secretions but has been increasingly implicated as a cause of genital ulcer disease [5]. HSV-2 has more typically been associated with genital ulcer disease and is transmitted by sexual contact. HSV infections are extremely common in women of reproductive age. Approximately 1.6 million new cases of genital herpes are acquired annually in the United States, and 22% of pregnant women have serologic evidence of infection with HSV-2 [6,7]. More than 2% of women seroconvert during their pregnancy, placing their infants at higher risk for devastating disease [8]. Neonatal HSV disease occurs in approximately 1 of 3200 deliveries, resulting in 1500 cases of neonatal HSV each year [9]. Neonatal HSV infection is quite often a devastating disease, and it is this fact that underlies the urgency of identification and prevention efforts among pregnant women. HSV infection presents in the neonate as disseminated disease (involving multiple visceral organs), central nervous system (CNS) disease (with or without skin lesions), or localized disease (skin, eye, and mouth [SEM]). Mortality is high for disseminated disease (29%), lower for CNS disease (as low as 4% in recent years), and almost nonexistent for SEM disease with the advent of effective antiviral therapy [9]. Morbidity remains severe for CNS disease even in the era of acyclovir treatment, with only 31% of affected neonates demonstrating normal neurologic development [9]. Thus, prevention of transmission of HSV to the neonate remains an important goal.

Neonatal herpes occurs primarily as a result of exposure of an infant to the infected maternal genital tract around the time of delivery; with the cervix as the site of highest viral replication [10,11]. HSV transmission to the neonate in the perinatal period accounts for 85% of cases, with the remainder occurring by means of intrauterine or postnatal acquisition [8]. The risk for transmitting HSV to the neonate is highest when a pregnant woman acquires primary HSV infection during the third trimester. Transmission after primary HSV infection late in gestation has been estimated at 50%, compared with the risk for transmission in cases of recurrent HSV of 3% or less [12–14]. Discriminating primary from recurrent genital herpes disease is not trivial, however, making individual risk assessment in individual cases challenging. Greater than 75% of neonates born with HSV infection are born to women who are completely asymptomatic at delivery, which makes recognition and prevention efforts problematic [15]. The current standard of care for prevention of transmission of HSV to the neonate is to perform cesarean delivery for any woman in whom active genital ulcerative lesions typical of HSV are present on presentation in labor and for those who have a history of HSV and present with prodromal symptoms suggestive of a recurrence [16]. This standard of care has been in place for several years and remains so even with advances in HSV diagnostic and therapeutic options. Brown and colleagues [10] provided compelling evidence supporting the efficacy of cesarean delivery in reducing neonatal transmission of HSV in a prospective study of more than 58,000 pregnant women. In this study, 202 pregnant women were culture-positive for HSV at the time of presentation in labor. Among infants delivered by these women, 5% (10 of 202) developed neonatal HSV infection. One percent (1 of 85) of these infections occurred among infants delivered by means of cesarean section versus 7.7% (9 of 117) who were delivered vaginally, demonstrating that cesarean delivery significantly reduced transmission of HSV from mother to child ($P = .047$; 95% confidence interval [CI]: 0.02–1.08). This is the only prospective study demonstrating the efficacy of cesarean delivery in the prevention of neonatal HSV infection.

The need for cesarean delivery to prevent neonatal acquisition can be diminished through interventions that prevent maternal genital herpes acquisition in the third trimester by HSV-seronegative mothers. One strategy that is not universally accepted involves defining the risk for primary HSV infection through serologic screening of pregnant women and their partners [10]. Women who are HSV-negative but with HSV-seropositive partners can be counseled to use condoms or avoid sexual contact during this critical period. For women with known recurrent genital herpes, some practitioners prescribe antiviral prophylaxis beginning at 36 weeks of gestation. Randomized controlled clinical trials [17–22] have shown that antiviral therapy administered to women late in pregnancy reduces the episodes of recurrent herpes at delivery and, ultimately, limits the number of cesarean deliveries performed for this indication. Table 1 details the findings of six major randomized controlled trials conducted in the United States and Europe assessing the role of suppressive therapy in limiting HSV recurrences and the necessity for cesarean delivery. In the largest of these trials, administration of valacyclovir beginning at 36 weeks of gestation was demonstrated to reduce clinical HSV recurrences and reduced the number of women with clinical genital HSV at delivery by 70% [17]. Shedding of HSV at delivery was substantially lower in valacyclovir recipients as well (2% versus 24% in the placebo group). These data support the utility of antiviral prophylaxis in diminishing the need for cesarean delivery for clinical HSV recurrences.

Currently, the use of antiviral prophylaxis in those individuals with recurrent HSV infection remains controversial. The American College of Obstetricians and Gynecologists (ACOG) has not recommended that this practice be universally adopted. One concern regarding suppressive antiviral therapy is whether symptomatic recurrences may be replaced by asymptomatic shedding, which would potentially place an infant at greater risk for HSV acquisition at the time of delivery. Scott and colleagues [20] discovered that although there was a significant decrease in the presence of clinical genital lesions (6% versus 14%) with suppressive acyclovir therapy versus placebo, respectively, there was no difference in subclinical shedding (0%

Table 1
The efficacy of antiviral prophylaxis versus placebo in preventing HSV recurrence and the need
for cesarean delivery

Study	Women enrolled (n)	Intervention (n)	Recurrence at delivery (%)	P/OR	Cesarean deliveries for HSV (%)	P/OR
Sheffield et al [17]	350	Valacyclovir (178)	4%	P = .009	4%	P = .009
		Placebo (172)	13%	OR = 0.30	13%	OR = 0.30
Andrews et al [18]	112	Valacyclovir (57)	5.3%	P = .121	5.3%	P = .199
		Placebo (55)	14.6%		12.7%	
Scott et al [20]	234	Acyclovir (116)	6%	P = .046	7%	P = .172
		Placebo (118)	14%	OR = 0.40	12%	OR = 0.54
Braig et al [21]	288	Acyclovir (167)	0%	P = .0003	0%	P = .01
		Placebo (121)	12.4%		12.4%	
Brocklehurst et al [19]	63	Acyclovir (31)	6%	OR = 0.30	13%	OR = 0.44
		Placebo (32)	18.7%		25%	
Scott et al [22]	46	Acyclovir (21)	0%	P = .02	0%	P = .02
		Placebo (25)	36%	OR = 0.04	36%	OR = 0.04

Abbreviation: OR, odds ratio.
Data from Refs. [17–22].

versus 3%); therefore clinical lesions were not replaced by asymptomatic shedding of HSV. A second concern relates to toxicity to the neonate. Although no adverse effects of treatment have been observed in the neonates involved in trials of prophylaxis, further investigation is warranted to establish the safety profile of antenatal acyclovir exposure [17–22]. Acyclovir has been noted to induce neutropenia during treatment trials for neonatal HSV [23,24], and similar toxicity could potentially be seen if acyclovir or valacyclovir is widely used from 36 weeks of gestation until the time of delivery.

Cost-benefit analyses have indicated that women with recurrent genital herpes and lesions at delivery who undergo cesarean delivery not only have increased maternal morbidity and mortality when compared with the same women who deliver vaginally but incur a substantial financial burden [20,25]. An analysis performed in the early 1990s confirmed that this practice resulted in greater than 1580 excess cesarean deliveries and cost $2.5 million per case of neonatal herpes prevented in contrast to women who underwent cesarean section for episodes of primary HSV, which resulted in only 9 excess cesarean sections for each case of neonatal herpes prevented [25]. Randolph and colleagues [26] undertook a study to compare the cost-effectiveness of using acyclovir prophylaxis late in pregnancy compared with performing a cesarean delivery for recurrent genital HSV lesions as a preventative measure for neonatal HSV transmission. These investigators concluded that acyclovir prophylaxis administered late in pregnancy in women who have genital HSV recurrence would prevent more neonatal HSV infection and be more cost-effective than cesarean delivery alone.

In summary, active genital HSV lesions at the time of presentation in labor remain a strong indication for cesarean delivery, and those with known recurrent HSV presenting with a prodromal illness suggesting recurrence should also be delivered by cesarean section. Antiviral prophylaxis late in gestation for women with recurrent HSV is likely to reduce the need for cesarean delivery but has not yet become universally accepted.

HIV-1

HIV-1 is the retrovirus responsible for the pandemic of AIDS. More than 2000 children worldwide are infected with HIV through mother-to-child transmission (MTCT) each day, for an astonishing total of approximately 750,000 children per year [27,28]. MTCT is the primary means by which young children become infected with HIV [29]. An increasing proportion of infants with perinatal HIV are born to women who acquire HIV infection during their pregnancy [30]. In the absence of any intervention, the risk for MTCT is approximately 15% to 30%, with rates increasing to as high as 30% to 45% when prolonged breastfeeding is taken into account [31]. In 1994, the Pediatric AIDS Clinical Trials Group (PACTG) 076 trial [29] established that administration of the antiretroviral agent zidovudine (AZT) to HIV-infected mothers during pregnancy and delivery and to their neonates for 6 weeks after birth reduced the risk for perinatal HIV transmission from 25.5% to 8.3%. There seems to be a benefit of antiretroviral therapy initiated within hours of birth on preventing neonatal infection even if prophylaxis before delivery has not occurred, although this effect is more modest [32]. Interventions to reduce the risk for MTCT focus primarily on a three-arm regimen of antiretroviral prophylaxis (during the prenatal, intrapartum, and neonatal periods), elective cesarean section, and avoidance of breastfeeding [28,33]. MTCT rates of less than 2% have been reported in countries in which all three arms are effectively implemented [28,34].

MTCT of HIV occurs most commonly during the intrapartum period, with approximately two thirds of transmission occurring during delivery and one third during gestation [32]. Postulated mechanisms by which this may occur are (1) maternal blood transfusion to the fetus during labor, (2) ascending infection after rupture of membranes, and (3) direct contact with infected secretions or blood from the maternal genital tract [32,33]. Kourtis and colleagues [32] proposed that approximately 50% of MTCT occurs during the process of placental separation from the uterine wall, an event that begins days before delivery, with another third occurring during active labor and delivery. Intrauterine transmission before the onset of labor, sometimes early in gestation, occurs in a few cases, as indicated by those infants with detectable HIV nucleic acid in their early days of life and by the isolation of virus from aborted fetuses early in gestation [35].

It has been postulated that the mode by which an infant is delivered may have effects on the immune system that may influence susceptibility to HIV infection. Before the onset of labor, the fetus resides in a sterile environment with an immune system that is kept at bay. Studies have found that neonates have lower levels of cellular activation with fewer memory T cells and B lymphocytes than adults [36]. During the labor process, immune activation occurs secondary to antigen exposure and rupture of membranes. Therefore, activated CD4 T lymphocytes should be more susceptible to infection with HIV and lead to increased replication of the virus [37]. Bernstein and colleagues [36] refuted this theory by comparing activation of fetal lymphocytes of infants born by means of normal spontaneous vaginal delivery (NSVD) with those born by means of elective cesarean delivery (defined as occurring before rupture of membranes [ROM] or onset of labor). Fetal lymphocyte activation was comparable in both groups, and there was no significant difference in susceptibility to HIV infection, regardless of the mode of delivery. Rather than immune activation, exposure to infected blood and genital secretions is likely to explain the increased risk to the infant of passing through the birth canal.

Several studies have evaluated the effect of elective cesarean delivery on the risk for perinatal transmission of HIV to an infant born to an infected mother [27]. Early observational studies failed to demonstrate a protective effect of cesarean delivery consistently [38,39]. Results from a prospective randomized trial undertaken to address this issue were reported by the European Mode of Delivery Collaboration in 1999 [40]. All women included in the study had a confirmed diagnosis of HIV infection and were randomized to undergo cesarean delivery or vaginal delivery at 38 weeks of gestation. Both groups were similar in terms of baseline characteristics. Only 1.8% (3 of 170) of the infants who were delivered by means of cesarean section were ultimately infected with HIV compared with 10.5% (21 of 200) who were delivered vaginally ($P < .001$). Elective cesarean delivery in this study reduced the risk for vertical transmission by 80%. This breakthrough study, in conjunction with results from prior observational studies, highlights the fact that elective cesarean delivery can significantly reduce the risk for MTCT of HIV when compared with alternate modes of delivery (Table 2) [34,40–42]. During the same year this study was published, the International Perinatal HIV Group [33] performed a meta-analysis of 15 prospective cohort studies conducted in the United States and Europe, evaluating the effects of elective cesarean delivery on the vertical transmission of HIV. After adjusting for covariates (receipt of antiretroviral therapy, maternal stage of disease, and infant birth weight), transmission rates were decreased by approximately 50% by elective cesarean delivery compared with all other modes of delivery (transmission rate: 19% versus 10% for cesarean delivery [odds ratio (OR) = 0.43; 95% CI: 0.33–0.56]). It should be noted, however that these studies were performed before the widespread use of the powerful combination antiretroviral therapy regimens that are presently the standard of care. The extremely effective medical regimens available for reducing MTCT drastically alter the risk-benefit equation for performing cesarean

Table 2
European mode of delivery collaborations: MTCT of HIV infection according to mode of delivery

Year	Mother-child pairs (n)	Mode of delivery	No. deliveries	No. children infected (%)	P
1994	1254	Vaginal	946	127 (17.6%)	NR
		Cesarean section	308	28 (11.7%)	
1999	370	Vaginal	200	21 (10.5%)	P<.001
(RCT)		Cesarean section	170	3 (1.8%)	
1999	347	Vaginal (+emergent cesarean section)	264	52 (20%)	P<.001
		Elective cesarean section	83	4 (5%)	
2005	1571	Vaginal	369	24 (6.5%)	P<.001
		Emergent cesarean section	239	6 (2.5%)	
		Elective cesarean section	971	16 (1.6%)	

Abbreviations: NR, not reported; RCT, randomized controlled trial.
Data from Refs. [34,40–42].

delivery to reduce HIV transmission. The risk for intrapartum transmission of HIV is proportional to the viral load of the mother [43,44]; thus, the added benefit of performing cesarean delivery at the lowest viral load levels or in those patients who have undetectable plasma virus is not certain. In recognition of this, the ACOG has stated that for pregnant HIV-infected women with viral loads greater than 1000 copies/mL, elective cesarean delivery before the rupture of membranes is recommended [45]. If the viral load is less than 1000 copies/mL, data were deemed insufficient to demonstrate a clear benefit. A recent review of MTCT among participants in the Agence Nationale de Recherche sur le SIDA (ANRS) French Perinatal Cohort confirmed that for those women with viral loads less than 400 copies/mL, there was no significant difference in rates of transmission by mode of delivery [46].

Surgical complications may be higher for HIV-infected women than for otherwise healthy women undergoing elective cesarean delivery. An observational study found that HIV-infected women undergoing cesarean delivery had higher rates of postpartum endometritis, sepsis, requirement for blood transfusion, pneumonia, and death [47]. HIV-infected women not taking antiretroviral therapy and those with significant immunosuppression demonstrate higher postoperative morbidity [48,49]. Elective cesarean delivery is associated with lower rates of infectious complications than emergent cesarean delivery, however, and most adverse events in HIV-infected women undergoing elective cesarean delivery as recommended by ACOG guidelines are minor. A Cochrane database review on this topic concluded that although risks were higher among HIV-infected women undergoing elective cesarean delivery than those delivering vaginally, they were significantly less than the risks associated with nonelective cesarean delivery. This review found that elective cesarean delivery was an effective means of reducing MTCT for those with detectable viral loads [27].

In summary, elective cesarean delivery is an effective means of reducing the rate of MTCT of HIV for women presenting without ideal control of viral replication. For those on highly active antiretroviral therapy who have undetectable or low viral loads, the added benefit of cesarean delivery is not established and is probably negligible.

Hepatitis C virus

Hepatitis C Virus (HCV) is a single-stranded RNA virus of the Flaviviridae family that is transmitted through exposure to infected blood, by sexual contact, or from mother to infant. HCV is the most common chronic blood-borne infection in the United States, with approximately 30,000 new cases diagnosed each year [50]. HCV currently is the leading cause of chronic liver disease in the United States and is also the leading cause of liver failure leading to transplantation [51]. Eighty-five percent of individuals infected with HCV develop chronic infection, which may progress to cirrhosis, end-stage liver disease, and hepatocellular carcinoma [52]. The magnitude of this problem is therefore large, and efforts to prevent transmission could potentially be of great benefit. Unlike HSV or HIV, however, there is little evidence favoring cesarean delivery for prevention of HCV transmission to the neonate.

The prevalence of HCV among pregnant women ranges from 1% to 5% [50]. Rates of HCV seropositivity are considerably higher among HIV-positive pregnant women [53]. Because screening of blood products has virtually eliminated transfusion as a major route of transmission of HCV, transmission from mothers to their neonates has emerged as an important mode of HCV transmission [50,54]. HCV transmission from mother to child can occur in utero or intrapartum. A study from the European Pediatric Hepatitis C Virus Network demonstrated that 31% of HCV-infected children were polymerase chain reaction (PCR)-positive within the first 3 days of life, indicating that they acquired infection in utero [55]. These investigators suggested that even higher numbers (up to one half of children studied) may have been infected in utero but simply had viral loads lower than the limit of detection at early time points. This high rate of intrauterine transmission suggests that the benefit of cesarean section in overall transmission rates is limited at best. The overall risk for MTCT of HCV is approximately 5% [56,57]. The presence of maternal viremia is a clear indicator of increased risk for vertical transmission. Generally speaking, the higher the maternal RNA level, the higher is the chance of transmission [58–61]. Maternal coinfection with HIV is also strongly associated with increased risk for transmission [50,54,62,63]. Finally, a history of maternal intravenous drug abuse and associated placental damage seems to increase the risk for vertical HCV transmission [64,65].

The mode of delivery has not been proved to affect vertical transmission rates of HCV [55,64,66,67]. The current standard of care in the United

States does not support the use of elective cesarean delivery for the purpose of preventing MTCT of HCV. There have been no randomized controlled trials to address the utility of cesarean delivery for this purpose; thus, the data arguing either way are weak. A recent Cochrane database review concluded that observational studies were generally not supportive of cesarean delivery to prevent HCV transmission but that the lack of randomized trials prevents a complete evaluation of the question [67].

The issue may not be quite so clear-cut with HIV/HCV-coinfected pregnant women. Schackman and colleagues [63] performed a case-based analysis and concluded that elective cesarean section would provide clinical benefits to infants at a reasonable cost for women who were HIV/HCV coinfected and had suppressed HIV RNA but had detectable HCV RNA levels. Elective cesarean sections performed for women HIV/HCV coinfected with suppressed HIV RNA but detectable HCV RNA prevented 45 vertical HCV transmissions per 1000 deliveries and increased maternal mortality by one death per 100,000 deliveries. These investigators concluded that of the approximately 2000 deliveries that occur annually to HIV/HCV-coinfected women in the United States, elective cesarean sections could potentially prevent 90 vertical HCV transmissions per year while incurring the risk for one additional maternal death every 50 years [63]. On the contrary, Marine-Barjoan and colleagues [54] demonstrated that infants born to mothers coinfected with HIV and HCV did not display a significant difference in HCV MTCT when delivered vaginally (7 of 134) or by means of caesarean section (5 of 80). Furthermore, no MTCT was observed in infants of mothers who had undetectable HCV viral loads at the time of delivery. The European Pediatric Hepatitis C Virus Network reported an HCV perinatal transmission rate of 6.2% and also found no protective effect of elective cesarean section delivery versus vaginal delivery [66,68]. Although HIV/HCV-coinfected women transmitted HCV to their infants more frequently than women with solitary HCV infection in this study, these results did not achieve statistical significance. Taken together, the data suggest that women should not be offered elective cesarean sections in the hopes of avoiding HCV transmission. At the current time, the standard of care for HIV/HCV-coinfected women is to make judgments regarding elective cesarean delivery based on HIV indications and not to perform cesarean delivery for the purpose of preventing HCV transmission in individuals who have undetectable HIV viral loads.

Cesarean delivery for prevention of transmission of other viral agents

Other viral agents are capable of transmission through the infected birth canal. Hepatitis B virus (HBV) is a blood-borne virus that is commonly transmitted perinatally. Approximately 20% to 30% of infants born to HBV-positive mothers become HBV-positive in early infancy. One study from Taiwan suggested that cesarean section combined with hepatitis B immunization is advisable to prevent transmission to infants of mothers who are chronic

HBV carriers with high serum HBV loads [69]. Cesarean delivery plays no role in modern management of the HBV-infected pregnant woman, however. The availability of effective active and passive immunoprophylaxis (hepatitis B vaccine and hepatitis B immune globulin) has negated consideration of cesarean section for this purpose.

Human papillomaviruses (HPVs) are sexually transmitted DNA viruses that commonly inhabit the female genital tract and are associated with cervical cancer, juvenile laryngeal polyposis, and condyloma acuminatum. The HPV 16 and 18 infection rate of infants born vaginally was higher than that seen in infants born by cesarean delivery (51.4% versus 27.3%; $P = .042$) [70]. There is considerable evidence for transplacental transmission of HPV, however, and there is no recommendation to perform cesarean delivery for consideration of preventing HPV-associated disease [71].

Considerations regarding perinatal transmission of bacterial diseases

The Group B streptococcus (GBS) is the most frequent cause of neonatal sepsis in the United States [72]. Between 10% and 30% of women in the United States are colonized with GBS at any given time [73]. Approximately 50% of infants who are born to woman colonized with GBS become colonized with GBS on their skin and mucosal surfaces, simply as a result of passage though the birth canal or from GBS ascending from the birth canal into the amniotic fluid. Approximately 1% to 2% of these colonized infants then go on to develop early-onset GBS sepsis. The risk for developing early-onset GBS sepsis is decreased by cesarean delivery [74]. Elective cesarean delivery could theoretically be used as an intervention to influence the incidence of GBS. There are several reasons why this is not a serious consideration. First, the high incidence of colonization and low overall attack rate would make the costs and risks high for the number of lives affected. More directly, however, there is already an effective noninvasive strategy to decrease neonatal sepsis using intrapartum antimicrobial prophylaxis (IAP). The wide applicability and low cost of IAP make consideration of cesarean delivery for this purpose moot. The authors note that the institution of universal screening and IAP has been quite successful at decreasing the incidence of invasive GBS disease, although further progress is needed [75]. As with GBS, other bacteria causing neonatal sepsis are commonly acquired through the birth canal but cause invasive disease at an even lower incidence than GBS. There is no indication for cesarean delivery for prevention of neonatal colonization with any of these bacterial organisms.

Summary

Cesarean delivery can prevent transmission of a limited number of infectious agents from mother to infant. HSV and HIV are the primary pathogens for which cesarean delivery should be contemplated. Pregnant women with active genital lesions or with known HSV infection and a prodromal illness consistent with recurrence at the time of presentation in labor should undergo cesarean delivery. Pregnant women who are HIV infected and have detectable viremia (> 1000 copies/mL) should be counseled regarding the potential benefits of cesarean delivery as an adjunct to antiretroviral therapy. HCV is a growing problem globally and can be transmitted intrapartum, but there is insufficient evidence supporting cesarean delivery as a means of reducing transmission to the infant. Overall, maternal infections represent a small proportion of the medical indications for cesarean delivery and are not a major cause of the increasing number of elective cesarean deliveries observed in recent years.

References

[1] Miesnik S, Reale B. A review of issues surrounding medically elective cesarean delivery. J Obstet Gynecol Neonatal Nurs 2007;36:605–15.

[2] Hamilton BE, Martin JA, Ventura SJ. Births: preliminary data for 2005. Hyattsville (MD): National Center for Health Statistics; 2006.

[3] Menacker F. Trends in cesarean rates for first births and repeat cesarean rates for low-risk women: United States, 1990–2003. Natl Vital Stat Rep 2005;54:1–8.

[4] Bettes BA, Coleman VH, Zinberg S, et al. Cesarean delivery on maternal request. Obstet Gynecol 2007;109:57–66.

[5] Roberts CM, Pfister JR, Spear SJ. Increasing proportion of herpes simplex virus type 1 as a cause of genital herpes infection in college students. Sex Transm Dis 2003;30:797–800.

[6] Brown ZA, Selke S, Zeh J, et al. The acquisition of herpes simplex virus during pregnancy. N Engl J Med 1997;337:509–15.

[7] Schillinger JA, Xu F, Sternberg MR, et al. National seroprevalence and trends in herpes simplex virus type 1 in the United States, 1976–1994. Sex Transm Dis 2004;31:753–60.

[8] Brown Z. Preventing herpes simplex virus transmission to the neonate. Herpes 2004;11: 175–86.

[9] Kimberlin D. Herpes simplex virus infections of the newborn. Semin Perinatol 2007;31: 19–25.

[10] Brown Z, Wald A, Morrow R, et al. Effect of serologic status and cesarean delivery on transmission rates of herpes simplex virus from mother to infant. JAMA 2003;289:203–9.

[11] Nahmias A, Josey W, Naib Z, et al. Perinatal risk associated with maternal genital herpes simplex virus infection. Am J Obstet Gynecol 1971;110:825–36.

[12] Brown Z, Benedetti J, Selke S, et al. Asymptomatic maternal shedding of herpes simplex virus at the onset of labor: relationship to preterm labor. Obstet Gynecol 1996;87:483–8.

[13] Yeager AS, Arvin AM, Urbani LJ, et al. Relationship of antibody to outcome in neonatal herpes simplex virus. Infect Immun 1980;29:532–8.

[14] Prober CG, Corey L, Brown Z, et al. The management of pregnancies complicated by genital infections with herpes simplex virus. Clin Infect Dis 1992;15:1031–8.

[15] Peng J, Krause P, Kresch M. Neonatal herpes simplex virus infection after cesarean section with intact amniotic membranes. J Perinatol 1996;16:397–9.

[16] ACOG practice bulletin. Management of herpes in pregnancy. Number 8, October 1999. Clinical management guidelines for obstetrician-gynecologists. Int J Gynaecol Obstet 2000;68:165–73.

[17] Sheffield JS, Hill JB, Hollier LM, et al. Valacyclovir prophylaxis to prevent recurrent herpes at delivery. Obstet Gynecol 2006;108:141–7.

[18] Andrews WW, Kimberlin DF, Whitley R, et al. Valacyclovir therapy to reduce recurrent genital herpes in pregnant women. Am J Obstet Gynecol 2006;194:774–81.

[19] Brocklehurst P, Kinghorn G, Carney O, et al. A randomized placebo controlled trial of suppressive acyclovir in late pregnancy in women with recurrent genital herpes infection. Br J Obstet Gynaecol 1998;105:275–80.

[20] Scott LL, Hollier LM, McIntire D, et al. Acyclovir suppression to prevent recurrent genital herpes at delivery. Infect Dis Obstet Gynecol 2002;10:71–7.

[21] Braig S, Luton D, Sibony O, et al. Acyclovir prophylaxis in late pregnancy prevents recurrent genital herpes and viral shedding. Eur J Obstet Gynecol Reprod Biol 2001;96: 55–8.

[22] Scott LL, Sanchez PJ, Jackson GL, et al. Acyclovir suppression to prevent cesarean delivery after first-episode genital herpes. Obstet Gynecol 1996;87:69–73.

[23] Kimberlin D, Powell D, Gruber W, et al. Administration of oral acyclovir suppressive therapy after neonatal herpes simplex virus disease limited to the skin, eyes and mouth: results of a phase I/II trial. Pediatr Infect Dis J 1996;15:247–54.

[24] Kimberlin DW, Lin CY, Jacobs RF, et al. Safety and efficacy of high-dose intravenous acyclovir in the management of neonatal herpes simplex virus infections. Pediatrics 2001;108: 230–8.

[25] Randolph AG, Washington AE, Prober CG. Cesarean delivery for women presenting with genital herpes lesions. Efficacy, risks, and costs. JAMA 1993;270:77–82.

[26] Randolph AG, Hartshorn RM, Washington AE. Acyclovir prophylaxis in late pregnancy to prevent neonatal herpes: a cost-effectiveness analysis. Obstet Gynecol 1996;88: 603–10.

[27] Read JS, Newell ML. Efficacy and safety of cesarean delivery for prevention of mother-to-child transmission of HIV-1. Cochrane Database Syst Rev 2005;(4):CD005479.

[28] Newell ML. Current issues in the prevention of mother-to-child transmission of HIV-1 infection. Trans R Soc Trop Med Hyg 2006;100:1–5.

[29] Connor EM, Sperling RS, Gelber R, et al. Reduction of maternal-infant transmission of human immunodeficiency virus type 1 with zidovudine treatment. N Engl J Med 1994; 331:1173–80.

[30] Jamieson DJ, Clark J, Kourtis AP, et al. Recommendations for human immunodeficiency virus screening, prophylaxis, and treatment for pregnant women in the United States. Am J Obstet Gynecol 2007;197(Suppl 3):S26–32.

[31] UNAIDS. Prevention of mother-to-child-transmission of HIV. Available at: http://www.unaids.org/en/PolicyAndPractice/Prevention/PMTCT. Accessed April 10, 2008.

[32] Kourtis AP, Bulterys M, Nesheim SR, et al. Understanding the timing of HIV transmission from mother to infant. JAMA 2001;285:709–12.

[33] International Perinatal HIV Group. The mode of delivery and the risk of vertical transmission of human immunodeficiency virus type 1. N Engl J Med 1999;340:977–87.

[34] European Collaborative Study. Mother-to-child transmission of HIV infection in the era of highly active antiretroviral therapy. Clin Infect Dis 2005;40:458–65.

[35] Kuhn L, Stein ZA, Thomas PA, et al. Maternal-infant HIV transmission and circumstances of delivery. Am J Public Health 1994;84:1110–5.

[36] Bernstein HB, Jackson RW, Anderson J, et al. The effect of elective cesarean delivery and intrapartum infection on fetal lymphocyte activation and susceptibility to HIV infection. Am J Obstet Gynecol 2002;187:1283–9.

[37] McCloskey TW, Cavaliere T, Bakshi S, et al. Immunophenotyping of T lymphocytes by three-color flow cytometry in healthy newborns, children, and adults. Clin Immunol Immunopathol 1997;84:46–55.

[38] Landesman SH, Kalish LA, Burns DN, et al. Obstetrical factors and the transmission of human immunodeficiency virus type 1 from mother to child. The Women and Infants Transmission Study. N Engl J Med 1996;334:1617–23.

[39] Simonds RJ, Steketee R, Nesheim S, et al. Impact of zidovudine use on risk and risk factors for perinatal transmission of HIV. Perinatal AIDS Collaborative Transmission Studies. AIDS 1998;12:301–8.

[40] The European Mode of Delivery Collaboration. Elective caesarean-section versus vaginal delivery in prevention of vertical HIV-1 transmission: a randomized clinical trial. Lancet 1999;353:1035–9.

[41] The European Collaborative Study. Caesarean section and risk of vertical transmission of HIV-1 infection. Lancet 1994;343:1464–7.

[42] The European Collaborative Study. Maternal viral load and vertical transmission of HIV-1: an important factor but not the only one. AIDS 1999;13:1377–85.

[43] Garcia PM, Kalish LA, Pitt J, et al. Maternal levels of plasma human immunodeficiency virus type 1 RNA and the risk of perinatal transmission. Women and Infants Transmission Study Group. N Engl J Med 1999;341:394–402.

[44] Mofenson LM, Lambert JS, Stiehm ER, et al. Risk factors for perinatal transmission of human immunodeficiency virus type 1 in women treated with zidovudine. Pediatric AIDS Clinical Trials Group Study 185 Team. N Engl J Med 1999;341:385–93.

[45] Committee on Obstetric Practice. ACOG committee opinion scheduled cesarean delivery and the prevention of vertical transmission of HIV infection. Number 234, May 2000 (replaces number 219, August 1999). Int J Gynaecol Obstet 2001;73:279–81.

[46] Warszawski J, Tubiana R, Le Chenadec J, et al. Mother-to-child HIV transmission despite antiretroviral therapy in the ANRS French Perinatal Cohort. AIDS 2008;22:289–99.

[47] Louis J, Landon MB, Gersnoviez RJ, et al. Perioperative morbidity and mortality among human immunodeficiency virus infected women undergoing cesarean delivery. Obstet Gynecol 2007;110:385–90.

[48] Maiques-Montesinos V, Cervera-Sanchez J, Bellver-Pradas J, et al. Post-cesarean section morbidity in HIV-positive women. Acta Obstet Gynecol Scand 1999;78:789–92.

[49] Rodriguez EJ, Spann C, Jamieson D, et al. Postoperative morbidity associated with cesarean delivery among human immunodeficiency virus-seropositive women. Am J Obstet Gynecol 2001;184:1108–11.

[50] Jain S, Goharkhay N, Saade G, et al. Hepatitis C in pregnancy. Am J Perinatol 2007;24: 251–6.

[51] Rustgi VK. The epidemiology of hepatitis C infection in the United States. J Gastroenterol 2007;42:513–21.

[52] Rakela J, Vargas HE, Hepatitis C. Magnitude of the problem. Liver Transpl 2002;8: S3–6.

[53] Thomas DL, Villano SA, Riester KA, et al. Perinatal transmission of hepatitis C virus from human immunodeficiency virus type 1-infected mothers. Women and Infants Transmission Study. J Infect Dis 1998;177:1480–8.

[54] Marine-Barjoan E, Berrebi A, Giordanengo V, et al. HCV/HIV co-infection, HCV viral load and mode of delivery: risk factors for mother-to-child transmission of hepatitis C virus. AIDS 2007;21:1811–5.

[55] Mok J, Pembrey L, Tovo PA, et al. When does mother to child transmission of hepatitis C virus occur? Arch Dis Child 2005;90:F156–60.

[56] Schwimmer JB, Balistreri WF. Transmission, natural history, and treatment of hepatitis C virus infection in the pediatric population. Semin Liver Dis 2000;20:37–46.

[57] Thomas SL, Newell ML, Peckham CS, et al. A review of hepatitis C virus (HCV) vertical transmission: risks of transmission to infants born to mothers with and without HCV viraemia or human immunodeficiency virus infection. Int J Epidemiol 1998;27: 108–17.

[58] Ceci O, Margiotta M, Marello F, et al. Vertical transmission of hepatitis C virus in a cohort of 2,447 HIV-seronegative pregnant women: a 24-month prospective study. J pediatr Gastroenterol Nutr 2001;33:570–5.

[59] Lin HH, Kao JH, Hsu HY, et al. Possible role of high-titer maternal viremia in perinatal transmission of hepatitis C virus. J Infect Dis 1994;169:638–41.

[60] Moriya T, Sasaki F, Mizui M, et al. Transmission of hepatitis C virus from mothers to infants: its frequency and risk factors revisited. Biomed Pharmacother 1995;49:59–64.

[61] Ohto H, Terazawa S, Sasaki N, et al. Transmission of hepatitis C virus from mothers to infants. The Vertical Transmission of Hepatitis C Virus Collaborative Study Group. N Engl J Med 1994;330:744–50.

[62] Gibb DM, Goodall RL, Dunn DT, et al. Mother-to-child transmission of hepatitis C virus: evidence for preventable peripartum transmission. Lancet 2000;356:904–7.

[63] Schackman BR, Oneda K, Goldie SJ. The cost-effectiveness of elective cesarean delivery to prevent hepatitis C transmission in HIV-coinfected women. AIDS 2004;18:1827–34.

[64] Resti M, Azzari C, Mannelli F, et al. Mother to child transmission of hepatitis C virus: prospective study of risk factors and timing of infection in children born to women seronegative for HIV-1. BMJ 1998;317:437–41.

[65] Mast E, Hwang L, Seto D, et al. Risk factors for perinatal transmission of hepatitis C virus (HCV) and the natural history of HCV infection acquired in infancy. J Infect Dis 2005;192: 1880–9.

[66] European Paediatric Hepatitis C Virus Network. A significant sex- but not elective cesarean section- effect on mother-to-child-transmission of hepatitis C infection. J Infect Dis 2005; 192:1872–9.

[67] McIntyre PG, Tosh K, McGuire W. Caesarean section versus vaginal delivery for preventing mother to infant hepatitis C virus transmission. Cochrane Database Syst Rev 2006;(4):CD005546. (Online).

[68] European Paediatric Hepatitis C Virus Network. Effects of mode of delivery and infant feeding on the risk of mother-to-child transmission of hepatitis C virus. Br J Obstet Gynaecol 2001;108:371–7.

[69] Lee SD, Lo KJ, Tsai YT, et al. Role of caesarean section in prevention of mother-infant transmission of hepatitis B virus. Lancet 1988;2:833–4.

[70] Tseng CJ, Liang CC, Soong YK, et al. Perinatal transmission of human papillomavirus in infants: relationship between infection rate and mode of delivery. Obstet Gynecol 1998;91: 92–6.

[71] Kosko JR, Derkay CS. Role of cesarean section in prevention of recurrent respiratory papillomatosis—is there one? Int J pediatr Otorhinolaryngol 1996;35:31–8.

[72] Hager WD, Schuchat A, Gibbs R, et al. Prevention of perinatal group B streptococcal infection: current controversies. J Perinat Med 2006;96:141–5.

[73] Renner RM, Renner A, Schmid S, et al. Efficacy of a strategy to prevent neonatal early-onset group B streptococcal (GBS) sepsis. J Perinat Med 2006;34:32–8.

[74] Bramer S, Van Wijk FH, Mol BW, et al. Risk indicators for neonatal early-onset GBS-related disease. A case-control study. J Perinat Med 1997;25:469–75.

[75] Centers for Disease Control and Prevention (CDC). Early-onset and late-onset neonatal group B streptococcal disease—United States, 1996–2004. MMWR Morb Mortal Wkly Rep 2005;54:1205–8.

ELSEVIER
SAUNDERS

CLINICS IN
PERINATOLOGY

Clin Perinatol 35 (2008) 421–435

Cesarean Section and the Outcome of Very Preterm and Very Low-Birthweight Infants

Michael H. Malloy, MD, MS[a,b,]*,
Snehal Doshi, MD, MSEd[a,b]

[a]*Department of Pediatrics, University of Texas Medical Branch, 301 University Boulevard, Galveston, TX 77555-0526, USA*
[b]*Division of Neonatology, University of Texas Medical Branch, Galveston, TX, USA*

Cesarean section has provided a life-saving form of delivery for pregnancies gone awry since first reported in ancient and medieval history. During that time period, however, the fetal life saved was at the expense of the mother's life [1]. With the advent of safe anesthesia and modern surgical techniques, delivery by cesarean section has become a more routine procedure to the extent that it has been used as the delivery method of choice for women who have had previous cesarean sections and a delivery method of convenience for some obstetricians and women who have low-risk pregnancies [1]. This is made apparent by examining the burgeoning rate of primary cesarean section in the United States among low-risk term pregnancies [2]. As a result, the life-preserving qualities of cesarean section for pregnancies at risk may be overlooked by the observation that among low-risk term pregnancies the risk for neonatal mortality is actually higher among infants delivered by cesarean section [3]. The reasons for this observation remain obscure.

The impact of cesarean section among extremely preterm and very low-birthweight infants lacks consensus. Some studies have suggested that this mode of delivery conveys advantages to survival, whereas others have suggested no such advantage but no additional risk above and beyond the risks associated with being born extremely preterm [4–14]. The reasons for the variability in results of these studies may be associated with analytic issues

* Corresponding author. Department of Pediatrics, University of Texas Medical Branch, 301 University Boulevard, Galveston, TX 77555-0526.
E-mail address: mmalloy@utmb.edu (M.H. Malloy).

0095-5108/08/$ - see front matter © 2008 Elsevier Inc. All rights reserved.
doi:10.1016/j.clp.2008.03.008
perinatology.theclinics.com

that may fail to take into account circumstances that confound the relationship between cesarean section and outcome in this population of extremely preterm infants. With the increasing rate of cesarean section reported among extremely preterm births in the United States, the question arises as to whether or not there is any justification for this increasing rate (Fig. 1).

The purpose of this review is to examine some of the analytic issues that confound the relationship between cesarean section and outcome in the population of extremely preterm infants, to review recent observations on neonatal mortality and cesarean section, to examine other outcomes relative to the mode of delivery, and to review the impact of cesarean section on maternal outcome.

Much of the data presented in this review comes from a recent analysis of United States Vital Statistics Linked Birth and Infant Death Certificate files for the years 2000 to 2003. A description of the methodologies used in that analysis is reported in the literature [15].

Analytic issues

Birthweight versus gestational age

A major confounding issue in analyzing outcomes among infants by using birthweight is the impact of being small for gestational age (SGA). Analyzing data by various birthweight intervals allows for the inclusion of SGA infants in each interval who have better outcomes. Thus, with the inclusion of SGA infants, the mortality for any given birthweight interval is reduced. Fig. 2 compares the neonatal mortality for the years 2000 to 2003 in the United States, as determined for 100-g intervals from 500 g through 1400 g, to the "untrimmed" neonatal mortality data for each gestational age from 22 weeks' gestation through 31 weeks' gestation ("trimmed" and "untrimmed" data discussed later). Through 28 weeks,

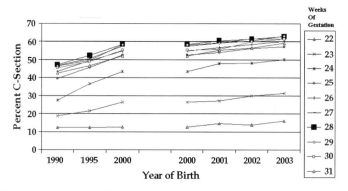

Fig. 1. Cesarean section rates (%) for very preterm infants by year and gestational age: United States 1990–2003.

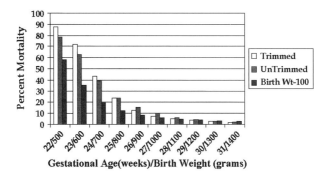

Fig. 2. Neonatal mortality by gestational age and 100-g birthweight intervals for trimmed and untrimmed data: United States 2000–2003.

neonatal mortality is considerably lower when examined by 100-g birthweight intervals compared with the gestational age equivalent. Although inclusion of SGA status in a multivariate analysis may diminish the SGA impact on mortality, as in most such analyses, such control is not absolute. Thus, a more conservative method of analysis of mortality is by examination by weeks of gestation.

Errors in gestational age calculation

One of the problems in working with any observational data, in particular vital statistics data, is the misclassification of gestational age. Although the National Center for Health Statistics, which is responsible for the collection and dissemination of United States Vital Statistics data, has designed an algorithm that attempts to screen out birthweights that are inconsistent with gestational age, the screening procedure ranges for a birthweight considered consistent with gestational age are broad [16]. Birthweights up to 2000 g are deemed acceptable for 22 to 23 weeks' gestation, up to 3000 g for 24 to 27 weeks', and up to 4000 g for 28 to 31 weeks'. These ranges are too inclusive to give a good understanding of the outcome among infants in this very immature gestational range. A method to get around the issue of gestational age misclassification is to trim away birthweights that fall outside specified ranges of weights for a particular gestational age.

Birthweight-trimming formulas for specific gestational ages

Formulas used to trim birthweights for specific gestational age intervals use the mode, mean, or median from the underlying birthweight distribution for a gestational age and set cutoff ranges around that central point based on observed or hypothetical normal distribution using 1 or 2 SDs as cutoff points or using inter-range intervals as cutoff points [17–20]. In the analyses presented in this article, the mode or most frequently occurring birthweight for each week of gestation was used and one half of the interquartile range on both sides of the mode were selected as cutoff points [15]. Although this trimming process diminished the number of births available at each gestation by approximately 50%, the resulting analysis gives a more conservative estimate of the impact of any intervention in a much smaller group of representative infants for a specific gestational age (Fig. 3). Through 24 weeks' gestation, the neonatal mortality in this trimmed dataset is higher than that among the untrimmed dataset (see Fig. 2).

Age of death

The selection of the age of death to examine as a primary outcome in evaluating cesarean section and vaginal deliveries among extremely preterm infants is important. Neonatal mortality (deaths occurring from the day of birth to 27 days of age) provides an overview of outcomes that may relate to the impact of the mode of delivery; however, it does not give the entire picture. The major impact of cesarean section is in the first day of life. From days 2 to 6, the percent mortality rate for infants born by cesarean section is higher as is the day 7 to day 27 percent mortality rate. The overall survival rate for cesarean sections, however, is higher for cesarean sections because of the much lower day 1 mortality rate associated with cesarean sections (this observation discussed later).

Complications of pregnancy and delivery

A long list of maternal medical conditions and labor and delivery complications that can affect pregnancy outcome adversely and that may be an indication for cesarean section must be taken into consideration when evaluating the impact of the mode of delivery on outcome. Among the population of extremely preterm infants, approximately 90% have some type of complication associated with the pregnancy (see Ref. [15] for list of complications considered in "adjusted" analyses). The goal of such an analysis in

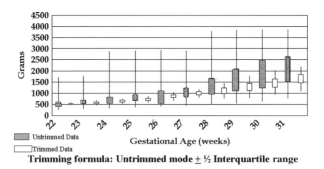

Fig. 3. Distribution of birthweight by gestation for untrimmed and trimmed data: United States 2000–2003.

which these complications are taken into account is to determine if the mode of delivery independent of these complications offers survival advantages. The most common means of controlling for these complications is through the use of multivariate logistic regression. Another way to approach this issue is to exclude women and pregnancies with these complications from the analysis. The problem with this latter approach is that because of the large proportion of pregnancies that deliver extremely preterm infants who have complications, the sample size for demonstrating an association between the mode of delivery and outcome may be too small to adequately power the analysis.

Mode of delivery comparison strategies

Comparison of the outcomes of primary cesarean sections to vaginal deliveries not associated with a previous cesarean section seems the most straightforward way to determine the impact of the mode of delivery on outcome. Repeat cesarean sections may involve recurrent conditions that could affect outcome and vaginal births after cesarean sections, which also may encounter increased risks. Primary cesarean sections at 25 weeks' gestation or less account for 85% or more of the cesarean sections performed except at 22 weeks' gestation when the percentage approaches 76%. Vaginal births after cesarean section account for less than 4% of vaginal births for gestational ages of 25 weeks or less in the United States for the years 2000 to 2003. Thus, a small proportion of births was excluded by dropping repeat cesarean sections and vaginal births after cesarean section.

Impact of cesarean section on mortality

Early mortality

As discussed previously, the percent mortality for vaginal delivery at 25 weeks' gestation or less on the first day of life is extremely high (41%) compared with infants delivered by cesarean section (12%). At 1 to 6 days, 7 to 27 days, and 28 to 354 days, the percent mortality for infants delivered by cesarean section exceeds vaginal delivery mortality. Nevertheless, the survival rate for the first year of life is greater for infants delivered by cesarean section (62% versus 38%). An argument can be made that the reason for the high mortality rate on the first day of life among infants delivered vaginally is that there is no attempt to resuscitate these infants. Whereas for infants delivered by cesarean section, it can be argued that if a decision is made to intervene with a cesarean section, it is more likely that some attempt would be made to resuscitate these infants. Thus, some attempt must be made to control for this possibility in an analysis of the impact on survival of the mode of delivery for these extremely preterm infants. This issue is discussed in the next section.

Neonatal mortality

Death from the first day of life through 27 days lends itself well as an outcome because 75% or more of deaths occurring in the first year of life occur during this period in infants less than 26 weeks' gestation (Fig. 4). In addition, it is more likely that a death occurring during this period might be related to an intervention at birth than a death occurring after 27 days of life. To derive an estimate of the risk for cesarean section for neonatal mortality compared with vaginal delivery independent of risk factors previously associated with neonatal mortality or the need for cesarean section, multivariate analysis is used to control or adjust for potentially confounding conditions. As part of the analytic process, multivariate models are developed and interactions or relationships between the primary risk factor of interest, in this case the mode of delivery, and other independent variables within the model are examined. Those interactions that turn up as significant require that separate models be run for each level of occurrence of the independent risk factor. In the analysis presented here, there is a significant interaction between the mode of delivery and gestational age. Thus, separate multivariate models were run for each week of gestation to develop a more valid estimate of the relationship between the mode of delivery and the outcome of interest, neonatal mortality, independent of other risk factors. The clinical implication of this interaction is that at each gestational age between 22 and 31 weeks' gestation there is a difference in the relationship between mode of delivery and the outcome.

Fig. 5 presents the raw and adjusted odds ratios (ORs) and 95% CIs for neonatal mortality for primary cesarean section compared with vaginal delivery. There are several points to note. First, there is little difference between the raw and adjusted ORs for most of the gestational ages examined. The only substantial difference is at 22 week' gestation where the adjusted OR is higher albeit still significantly less than 1.00. Also, the

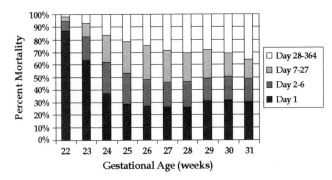

Fig. 4. Percent mortality by age at death and gestational age: United States 2000–2003 (trimmed data).

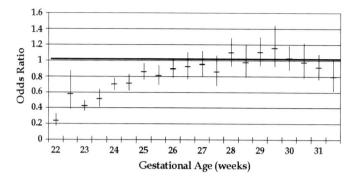

Fig. 5. Raw and adjusted ORs for neonatal mortality for primary cesarean section versus vaginal delivery: United States 2000–2003 (trimmed data). ORs adjusted for SGA, male, multiple birth, breech presentation, anomaly, 5-minute Apgar less than 4, presence of medical or labor-related complications, maternal age, maternal education, and race.

ORs for neonatal mortality are significantly reduced for gestational ages of 25 weeks or less, whereas for gestations of 26 or more weeks there is no significant reduction. This suggests that independent of other risk factors, primary cesarean section seems to provide some survival advantage to extremely preterm infants delivered at 25 weeks or less.

Another way to look at the issue of whether or not primary cesarean section offers survival advantages to preterm infants is to examine the outcome of infants who have various risk factors. Fig. 6 presents the ORs for neonatal mortality for high-risk pregnancies that included SGA infants, multiple births, breech presentations, infants who had congenital anomalies, pregnancies with medical or labor complications, and infants who had 5-minute Apgar scores less than 4. The ORs were adjusted for birthweight, maternal age, education, and race. These ORs demonstrate point estimates that all are

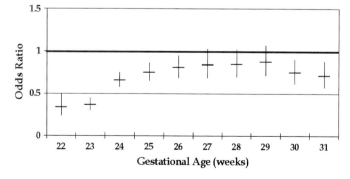

Fig. 6. Adjusted ORs for neonatal mortality for only high-risk pregnancies for primary cesarean section versus vaginal delivery: United States 2000–2003 (trimmed data). High-risk pregnancies included SGA infants, multiple births, breech presentations, anomalies, pregnancies with medical or labor complications, and infants who had 5-minute Apgar less than 4. ORs adjusted for birthweight, maternal age, education, and race.

below 1.00 with 95% CIs that exclude 1.0 for all gestations except 28 and 29 weeks. The implications for this analysis are that, as might be hoped and expected, that for extremely preterm infants born with significant risk factors primary cesarean section definitely offers survival advantages.

It may be argued that the reason for the apparent survival advantage of extremely preterm infants delivered by primary cesarean section at 25 weeks' gestation or less independent of other risk factors may be related to the likelihood that more resuscitative efforts are offered to these infants than to infants delivered vaginally. The argument is that if there is enough interest in putting a mother at risk with a cesarean section, a greater effort will be made to save the infant. In the following analysis, it is reasoned that if an infant was recorded as having received mechanical ventilation after birth, that was evidence that resuscitative efforts were undertaken. Fig. 7 shows the percentage of infants delivered vaginally and by primary cesarean section and the total percentage at each gestational age that received mechanical ventilation. For infants at gestational ages of 25 weeks or less, a greater percentage received mechanical ventilation if delivered by cesarean section. This is striking at 22 and 23 weeks' gestation. An analysis was undertaken examining only those infants who received mechanical ventilation adjusting the ORs for all risk factors. Fig. 8 shows a significant reduction in the ORs for neonatal mortality at 22 and 23 weeks. The equivalency of risk by mode of delivery for the reminder of the gestations may relate to issues having to do more with these infants' needs for mechanical ventilation than any impact of the mode of delivery.

In summary, when neonatal mortality is used as an endpoint, primary cesarean section does seem to offer survival advantages to infants born at 25 weeks or less independent of several known risk factors. The mechanism by which primary cesarean section offers this survival advantage is uncertain. Whether or not it relates simply to less trauma and the rigors a fetus may face going through labor is unknown. The ethical question that arises, however, is whether or not contributing to the survival of these extremely

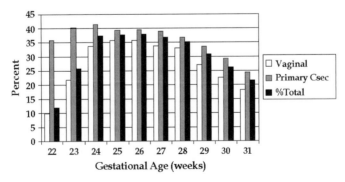

Fig. 7. Percent of infants receiving mechanical ventilation by mode of delivery: United States 2000–2003 (trimmed data).

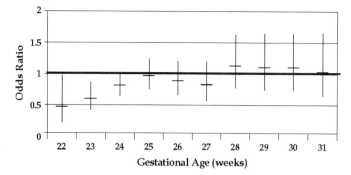

Fig. 8. Percent of infants receiving mechanical ventilation by mode of delivery: United States 2000–2003 (trimmed data). ORs adjusted for SGA, male, multiple birth, breech presentation, anomaly, 5-minute Apgar less than 4, presence of medical or labor-related complications, maternal age, maternal education, and race.

preterm infants, born at 25 weeks or less, who are at such high risk of neurodevelopmental problems is appropriate [21–24]. Informing parents of the risk for poor neurodevelopmental outcome, particularly for infants born at less than 24 weeks' gestation, should be part of the intrapartum decision-making process in which parents can participate [21].

Impact of cesarean section on other outcomes

Other major morbidities associated with the birth of extremely preterm infants include respiratory, neurologic, and intestinal. The relationship of these morbidities to the mode of delivery has been investigated to some degree for the first two. Below is a review of some of that literature and analyses using the trimmed dataset from the United States Vital Statistics Linked Birth and Infant Death Certificate files for 2000 to 2003 (discussed previously). The outcomes of particular interest relative to the mode of delivery are the occurrence of respiratory distress syndrome (RDS), intraventricular hemorrhage (IVH), asphyxia, and necrotizing enterocolitis (NEC).

Respiratory distress syndrome

Elective cesarean section has been observed to be associated with an increase risk for respiratory morbidity in term and near-term births [25–27]. The literature concerning the risk for respiratory morbidity relative to the mode of delivery in more immature infants, however, is not so clear cut. A Cochrane review of the issue of elective cesarean section versus expectant management for the delivery of small babies reported less RDS among infants delivered electively by cesarean section [28]. This was based, however, on only six studies that involved only 122 women who had been randomized to expectant management or elective cesarean. The impact of cesarean section on twin delivery outcomes of infants weighing less than 1500 g reported a higher prevalence of RDS among those twins delivered by cesarean (65.2% versus 42%) [29]. In a case-control study from Finland where the outcomes of 103 women who were delivered by cesarean section based on maternal or fetal indications were compared with the outcomes of 103 control patients who had no indications for cesarean section and were matched for gestational age, the relative risk for RDS was 1.4 (95% CI, 1.1–1.7).

The overall percentage of infants from 22 to 31 weeks' gestation reported to have hyaline membrane disease (HMD) in the trimmed Vital Statistics data for the years 2000 to 2003 was 12.8%. This seems to be a low estimate and probably represents under-reporting. Nevertheless, comparing the reporting of HMD/RDS by mode of delivery with adjustment for potential confounding risk factors suggests an increased risk for infants delivered by cesarean section before 25 weeks' gestation (Fig. 9). The remainder of the ORs suggests the risk is equivocal except for 30 weeks' gestation where there is a slight increase in risk for infants delivered by cesarean section. This analysis must be interpreted cautiously, however, because of the exceptionally low reporting of this condition in the vital statistics records.

In summary, based on the literature and the analysis presented in this article, the risk for respiratory morbidity seems to be at least moderately increased among very preterm infants delivered by cesarean section.

Intracranial/intraventricular hemorrhage

The issue of the association between the mode of delivery and the occurrence of intracranial hemorrhage or IVH has not been as well investigated as might be expected. Several studies have reported a protective effect of cesarean section for IVH or periventricular leukomalacia whereas others have not. Wilson-Costello and colleagues [22] reported a greater OR for intact

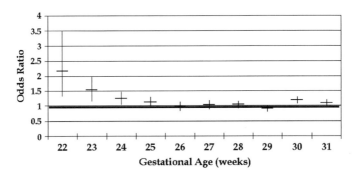

Fig. 9. Adjusted ORs for HMD cesarean versus vaginal delivery: United States 2000–2003 (trimmed data). ORs adjusted for SGA, male, multiple birth, breech presentation, anomaly, 5-minute Apgar less than 4, presence of medical or labor-related complications, maternal age, maternal education, and race.

neurodevelopmental survival free of severe IVH among infants born weighing less than 1000 g and delivered by cesarean section of 1.8 (95% CI , 1.35–2.46). Deulofeut and colleagues [30] found the risk for severe IVH to be higher among infants less than 751 g when delivered vaginally compared with cesarean delivery (OR 8.18; 95% CI, 1.58–42.2). In contrast, Malloy and colleagues [8] reported no significant protective effect of cesarean section for all grades of IVH when controlling for several risk factors among a group of infants weighing 501 to 1500 g. Wadhawan and colleagues [31] examined the effect of labor in conjunction with delivery by cesarean section and reported that although the incidence of severe IVH was lower among infants weighing less than 1000 g delivered by cesarean section with no labor (12.1% versus 23.3%), after controlling for several potentially confounding variables there were no significant differences that persisted. In a cohort study examining the effect of various types of antenatal glucocorticoid treatments on the occurrence of cystic periventricular leukomalacia in very preterm infants, delivery by cesarean section did not provide any protective effect in the adjusted logistic regression model (OR 0.83; 95% CI, 0.48–1.7) [32].

In summary, although it is appealing to believe that delivery by cesarean section is less traumatic to the very fragile extremely preterm brain, proof, at least as determined by examining for IVH or periventricular leukomalacia, is not convincing. Further examination of this issue using MRI studies for evidence of other neurologic lesions (ie, infarctions, ischemia, or white matter disruption) might provide more evidence.

Asphyxia

Although a somewhat difficult diagnosis to measure accurately, it is of interest as an outcome relative to the mode of delivery because of the potential impact the occurrence of this outcome may have on future neurodevelopmental outcome. In several studies where the diagnosis of asphyxia has been made based on cord blood base deficit measurements of greater than 12 mmol/L, cesarean section has been reported to be associated with a lower incidence of asphyxia, particularly for infants 22 to 25 weeks' gestation [33,34]. Alternately, Robilio and colleagues [35] reported a higher OR for asphyxia, based only on an International Classification of Diseases, Ninth Revision diagnosis, among very low-birthweight infants who had cephalic presentations delivered by cesarean section and who had been exposed to labor compared with cephalic presentation vaginal deliveries. The reason for these differences may be attributed to the inclusion of cesarean sections where the indication for intervention comes late after severe fetal asphyxia already has occurred. Low and coworkers' study graded the severity of the asphyxia and observed a lower frequency of mild and moderate asphyxia in cesarean deliveries [34]. Thus, the intervention (ie, cesarean section) may have been applied earlier avoiding severe asphyxia.

Although perhaps a poor proxy for asphyxia, using a 5-minute Apgar score of less than 4 may give some indication of the protective effect of the mode of delivery. An analysis of the trimmed 2000 to 2003 United States Vital Statistics data demonstrated an OR for an Apgar score less than 4 independent of other risk factors for gestations of 22 to 26 weeks to be significantly reduced for cesarean sections compared with vaginal deliveries; for gestations 27 to 30 weeks there were no significant differences by mode of delivery; and for gestations at 31 weeks the risk for a 5-minute Apgar score less than 4 was significantly increased for infants delivered by cesarean section (Fig. 10). These observations may be in line with the argument that cesarean section seems protective for asphyxia when applied earlier, before specific indications for intervention appear (eg, fetal distress). Thus, for the very early gestations of 22 to 26 weeks, cesarean sections may have been instigated before overt distress was apparent, giving rise to outcomes associated with fewer 5-minute Apgar scores less than 4.

In summary, there may be some evidence that cesarean sections may be associated with a diminished risk for asphyxia, particularly among the most immature infants.

Necrotizing enterocolitis

A relationship between the mode of delivery and the occurrence of intestinal disease, specifically NEC, does not seem biologically plausible. Only indirectly by virtue of a hypoxic incident does there seem likelihood of a relationship. The literature examining this relationship is limited. Uauy and colleagues [36], however, reported in a cohort of 2681 very low-birth-weight infants a decreased risk for NEC among infants delivered by cesarean section. No multivariate analysis correcting for potentially confounding variables was done. The investigators speculated, "prevention of hypoxic stress at delivery could be important in the prevention of NEC."

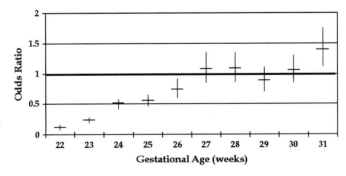

Fig. 10. Adjusted ORs for 5-minute Apgar score less than 4 cesarean versus vaginal delivery: United States 2000–2003 (trimmed data). ORs adjusted for SGA, male, multiple birth, breech presentation, anomaly, 5-minute Apgar less than 4, presence of medical or labor-related complications, maternal age, maternal education, and race.

Impact of cesarean section on maternal morbidity and mortality

The literature is replete with reports of increased risk for maternal morbidity and mortality with cesarean sections among term gestations, whether or not they are particularly low-risk planned cesarean sections or unplanned [37–42]. Despite some data suggesting that maternal mortality is not higher among women delivered by cesarean section compared with vaginal delivery in medium- and high-income countries or after adjustment for high-risk conditions, the health consequences of increasing cesarean section rates continue to be put forward [43–45]. Information on maternal morbidity and mortality risks in women delivered by cesarean section at very early gestations compared with women delivered vaginally is sorely lacking.

Summary

Based on recent analyses of data from the United States for the period 2000 to 2003, there seems to be some survival advantage associated with delivery of extremely preterm infants less than 25 weeks' gestation by cesarean section. This survival advantage must be weighed, however, against the extremely high risk for neurodevelopmental and respiratory morbidities observed among these infants. The consequences of performing a cesarean section on the immediate outcome of mothers and their future reproductive health also must be considered.

References

[1] Todman D. A history of caesarean section: from ancient world to the modern era. Aust N Z J Obstet Gynaecol 2007;47:357–61.

[2] Declercq E, Menacker F, MacDorman MF. Rise in "no indicated risk" primary cesareans in the United States, 1991–2001: cross sectional analysis. BMJ 2005;330:71–2.

[3] MacDorman MF, Declercq E, Menacker F, et al. Infant and neonatal mortality for primary cesarean and vaginal births to women with "no indicated risk", United States, 1998–2001 birth cohorts. Birth 2006;33:175–82.

[4] Stewart AL, Turcan DM, Rawlings G, et al. Prognosis for infants weighing 1000 grams or less at birth. Arch Dis Child 1977;52:97–104.

[5] Williams RL, Chen PM. Identifying the sources of the recent decline in perinatal mortality rates in California. N Engl J Med 1982;306:207–14.

[6] Sachs BP, McCarthy BJ, Rubin G, et al. Cesarean section: risk and benefits for mother and fetus. JAMA 1983;250:2157–9.

[7] Malloy MH, Rhoads GG, Schramm W, et al. Increasing cesarean section rates in very low-birth weight infants. JAMA 1989;262:1475–8.

[8] Malloy MH, Onstat L, Wright E. The national institute of child health and human development neonatal research network. Obstet Gynecol 1991;77:498–503.

[9] Holmgren PA, Hogberg U. The very preterm infant—a population-based study. Acta Obstet Gynecol Scand 2001;80:525–31.

[10] Lumley J. Method of delivery for the preterm infant. BJOG 2003;110(Suppl 20):88–92.

[11] Hakansson S, Farooqi A, Holmgren PA, et al. Proactive management promotes outcome in extremely preterm infants: a population-based comparison of two perinatal management strategies. Pediatrics 2004;114:58–64.

[12] Hogberg U, Hakansson S, Serenius F, et al. Extremely preterm cesarean delivery: a clinical study. Acta Obstet Gynecol Scand 2006;107:97–105.

[13] Lee HC, Gould JB. Survival advantage associated with cesarean delivery in very low birth weight vertex neonates. Obstet Gynecol 2006;107:97–105.

[14] Lee HC, Gould JB. Survival rates and mode of delivery for vertex preterm neonates according to small- or appropriate-for-gestational-age status. Pediatrics 2006;118:e1836. Available at: www.pediatrics.org/cgi/doi/10.1542/peds.2006-1327. Accessed March 28, 2008.

[15] Malloy MH. The impact of cesarean section on neonatal mortality among very preterm infants: United States 2000–2003. Pediatrics, in press.

[16] Division of Vital Statistics. Instruction manual part 12: computer edits for natality data, effective 1993. Vital statistics, data preparation. Hyattsville (MD): National Center for Health Statistics; 1995. Available at: www.cdc.gov/nchs/data/dvs/instr12.pdf.pp33-35. Accessed March 28, 2008.

[17] Williams RL. Appendix: final report for contract no. 75-5395 (MCH). In: Cunningham GC, Hawes WE, Madore C, editors. Intrauterine growth and neonatal risk in California. Santa Barbara (CA): University of California Community and Organization Research Institute; 1976. p. 16.

[18] Malloy MH, Hoffman HJ. Prematurity, sudden infant death syndrome, and age of death. Pediatrics 1995;96:454–71.

[19] Alexander GR, Himes JH, Kaufman RB, et al. Obstet Gynecol 1996;87:163–8.

[20] Arnold CC, Kramer MS, Hobbs CA, et al. Very low birth weight: a problematic cohort for epidemiological studies of very small or immature neonates. Am J Epidemiol 1991;134: 604–13.

[21] MacDonald H. The Committee on Fetus and Newborn. Perinatal care at the threshold of viability. Pediatrics 2002;110:1024–7.

[22] Wilson-Costello D, Friedman H, Minich N, et al. Improved neurodevelopmental outcomes of extremely low birth weight infants in 2000–2002. Pediatrics 2007;119:37–45.

[23] Tommiska V, Heinonen K, Lehtonen L, et al. No improvement in outcome of nationwide extremely low birth weight infant populations between 1996–1997 and 1999–2000. Pediatrics 2007;119:29–36.

[24] Marlow N, Hennessy EM, Bracewell MA, et al. Motor and executive function at 6 years of age after extremely preterm birth. Pediatrics 2007;120:793–803.

[25] Hansen AK, Wisborg K, Uldbjeerg N, et al. Elective caesarean section and respiratory morbidity in the term and near-term neonate. Acta Obstet Gynecol Scand 2007;86:389–94.

[26] Kolas T, Saugstad OD, Daltveit AK, et al. Planned cesarean versus planned vaginal delivery at term; comparison of newborn infant outcomes. Am J Obstet Gynecol 2006;195:1538–43.

[27] Jain L, Dudell GG. Respiratory transition in infants delivered by cesarean section. Semin Perinatol 2006;30:296–304.

[28] Grant A, Glazener CM. Elective caesarean section versus expectant management for delivery of the small baby. Cochrane Database Syst Rev 2001;(1):CD000078.

[29] Ziadeh SM, Badria LF. Effect of mode of delivery on neonatal outcome of twins with birthweight under 1500 g. Arch Gynecol Obstet 2000;264:128–30.

[30] Deulofeut R, Sola A, Lee B, et al. The impact of vaginal delivery in premature infants weighing less than 1,251 grams. Obstet Gynecol 2005;105:525–31.

[31] Wadhawan R, Vohr BR, Fanaroff AA, et al. Does labor influence neonatal and neurodevelopmental outcomes of extremely-low-birth-weight infants who are born by cesarean delivery? Am J Obstet Gynecol 2003;189:501–6.

[32] Baud O, Foix-L'Helias L, Kaminski M, et al. Antenatal glucocorticoid treatment and cystic periventricular leukomalacia in very premature infants. N Engl J Med 1999;341:1190–6.

[33] Hogberg U, Hakansson S, Serenius F, et al. Extremely preterm cesarean delivery: a clinical study. Acta Obstet Gynecol Scand 2006;85:1442–7.

[34] Low JA, Killen H, Derrick EJ. The prediction and prevention of intrapartum fetal asphyxia in preterm pregnancies. Am J Obstet Gynecol 2002;186:279–82.

[35] Robilio PA, Boe NM, Danielsen B, et al. Vaginal vs. cesarean delivery for preterm breech presentation of singleton infants in California: a population-based study. J Reprod Med 2007;52:473–9.

[36] Uauy RD, Fanaroff AA, Korones SB, et al. Necrotizing enterocolitis in very low birth weight infants: biodemographic and clinical correlates. J Pediatr 1991;119:630–8.

[37] Liu S, Liston RM, Joseph KS, et al. Maternal mortality and severe morbidity associated with low-risk planned cesarean delivery versus planned vaginal delivery at term. CMAJ 2007;176: 455–60.

[38] Villar J, Valladares E, Wojdyla D, et al. Caesarean delivery rates and pregnancy outcomes: the 2005 WHO global survey on maternal and perinatal health in Latin America. Lancet 2006;367:1819–29.

[39] Belizan JM, Cafferata ML, Althabe F, et al. Risks of patient choice cesarean. Birth 2006;33: 167–9.

[40] National Collaborating Centre for Women's and Children's Health. Commissioned by the national institute for clincal excellence. Caesarean Section Clinical Guideline. Available at: http://www.nice.org.uk/nicemedia/pdf/CG013NICEguidelines.pdf. Accessed March 28, 2008.

[41] Vadnais M, Sachs B. Maternal mortality with cesarean delivery: a literature review. Semin Perinatol 2006;30:242–6.

[42] Wax JR. Maternal request cesarean versus planned spontaneous vaginal delivery: maternal morbidity and short term outcomes. Semin Perinatol 2006;30:247–52.

[43] Althabe F, Sosa C, Belizan JM, et al. Cesarean section rates and maternal and neonatal mortality n low-, medium-, and high-income countries: an ecological study. Birth 2006;33: 270–7.

[44] Lydon-Rochelle M, Holt VL, Easterling TR, et al. Cesarean delivery and postpartum mortality among primiparas in Washington state, 1987–1996. Obstet Gynecol 2001;97: 169–74.

[45] Belizan JM, Althabe F, Cafferata ML. Health consequences of the increasing caesarean section rates. Epidemiology 2007;18:485–6.

ELSEVIER
SAUNDERS

CLINICS IN
PERINATOLOGY

Clin Perinatol 35 (2008) 437–454

Long-Term Neurologic Outcome of Infants Born by Cesarean Section

Ira Adams-Chapman, MD

*Developmental Progress Clinic, Emory University School of Medicine,
46 Jesse Hill Jr. Drive, Atlanta, GA 30303, USA*

When a physician decides to perform an operative delivery of an unborn fetus, the underlying goal is to optimize the outcome of the unborn infant or the mother. Prevention of neurologic injury to the fetus through skilled and attentive care during the peripartum period is designed to identify signs of fetal distress so that appropriate obstetric interventions can occur. The impact of mode of delivery on neurologic outcome has been heavily debated and varies depending on the clinical indication for cesarean delivery and the associated maternal and fetal conditions.

This review summarizes current knowledge of the impact of mode of delivery on long-term neurologic outcome.

Prematurity and mode of delivery

Perinatal mortality and mode of delivery

Interpretation of mortality and morbidity data for infants born at the edge of viability is difficult. The decision to intervene actively, from the obstetric and neonatal perspectives, is highly variable across centers [1,2]. Assessment of viability at various gestational ages (GAs) affects how we interpret rates of cesarean delivery and may affect neurodevelopmental outcome of surviving infants. Shankaran and colleagues [2] specifically evaluated the perinatal and neonatal management of extremely low birth weight (ELBW) neonates who died within 12 hours of life. Compared with those who died longer than 12 hours after birth or survived to hospital discharge, those who died within 12 hours were less likely to be delivered by cesarean birth and were less likely to have active delivery room

E-mail address: ira_adams-chapman@oz.ped.emory.edu

0095-5108/08/$ - see front matter © 2008 Elsevier Inc. All rights reserved.
doi:10.1016/j.clp.2008.03.001
perinatology.theclinics.com

resuscitation. Only 44% of those in the early death group were intubated in the delivery room compared with 92% of those in the late death and survivor group. Thus, these investigators believed that the high mortality rate among ELBW neonates who died within 12 hours was associated with a lack of perinatal and neonatal intervention that reflected the clinician's assessment of nonviability. Physicians often underestimate rates of survival and overestimate rates of neurodevelopmental impairment (NDI) [2–4]. Similarly, if the physician believes that the likelihood of intact survival is low, he or she is less likely to offer interventions, such as antenatal steroids, cesarean delivery for fetal distress, or transfer to a tertiary center, even though each of these has been associated with improved neurodevelopmental outcome [2–4]. The decision to manage the peripartum transition actively and intervene for signs of fetal distress is critical in prevention of fetal hypoxia and brain injury. Center-specific mortality and morbidity rates adjusted for GA should be provided to families facing imminent delivery of an extremely premature infant.

Understanding the risks associated with death also helps one to understand better the morbidity among surviving infants. Death and severe neurologic impairment are often combined for the purposes of analysis and interpretation of characteristics associated with poor neurologic outcome. The impact of mode of delivery on neonatal mortality is discussed in detail elsewhere in the text.

In an effort to evaluate the associations between mode of delivery and mortality, Lee and Gould [5] evaluated more than 8 million birth and death records over a 2-year period from data collected at the National Center for Health Statistics (NCHS) from singleton vertex-presenting infants. Fig. 1 graphically displays the birth weight–specific mortality rates based on mode of delivery. A multivariate logistic regression model was used to account for the impact of potential confounding variables. Cesarean delivery was associated with a 47% decrease in the very low birth weight (VLBW) neonatal mortality rate (odds ratio [OR] = 0.53, 95% confidence interval [CI]: 0.49–0.57). In contrast, among non-VLBW neonates, cesarean delivery was associated with a 62% increase in the neonatal mortality rate (OR = 1.62, 95% CI: 1.57–1.68). The protective advantage associated with cesarean delivery was most prominent for infants weighing less than 1300 g [5].

In a similar review, Jonas and Lumley [6] reported neonatal morbidity among a population-based cohort of 6164 VLBW infants weighing less than 1500 g in the Victorian Perinatal Registry. They excluded infants with malformations, elective repeat cesarean section, unknown delivery status, and GA less than 24 weeks and birth weight less than 500 g. Overall, VLBW infants delivered by cesarean section had a lower neonatal mortality rate compared with those delivered vaginally (10.4% versus 23.1%); however, after adjustment for GA, birth weight, birth year, birth hospital, labor, presentation, and indication for cesarean section, mode of delivery was no longer significant.

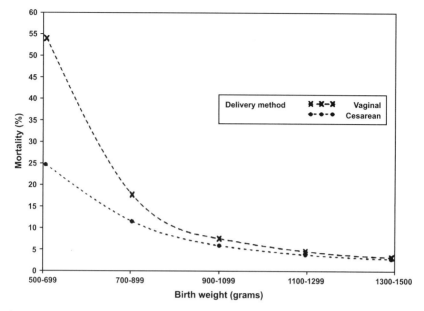

Fig. 1. Birth weight–specific mortality rates based on mode of delivery. (*From* Lee HC, Gould JB. Survival advantage associated with cesarean delivery in very low birth weight vertex neonates. Obstet Gynecol 2006;107:102; with permission).

Prematurity and intraventricular hemorrhage

Over the past 20 years, there have been dramatic advances in neonatal care resulting in improved neurodevelopmental outcome in premature infants; however, prematurity remains one of the most important causes of brain injury in the newborn. When one considers the fact that most intraventricular hemorrhage (IVH) occurs within the first 3 days of life [7], it is not surprising that many have sought to find associations between IVH and mode of delivery. Understanding this relation is important because premature infants with IVH are disproportionately represented among cases of neonatal brain injury and cerebral palsy (CP).

IVH is a serious complication of prematurity that has been associated with adverse long-term neurodevelopmental outcome and CP. The risk for hemorrhage is inversely related to GA and birth weight [8–10]. The risk for abnormal neurologic outcome is directly related to the severity of the hemorrhage [11–15].

Clinicians have speculated that the mechanical force and external pressure exerted on the compliant skull of the premature head during vaginal delivery increase the risk for brain injury and IVH [14,16,17]. This concern has resulted in a wide range of recommendations for mode of delivery in the preterm infant. In the early 1970s, many researchers advocated caesarean section for premature infants [18]. Others suggested that low forceps delivery resulted in a more controlled delivery of the fragile premature infant head [19,20]. Tejani and colleagues [21] provided some of the earliest data to support the current recommendation regarding mode of delivery in the preterm infant, which states that these infants should only be delivered by cesarean section if there are obstetric indications.

In 1987, Tejani and colleagues [21] performed a retrospective analysis of 280 preterm infants and found no difference in the risk for IVH based on mode of delivery. Similar findings have been reported in several recent reports [22–24], including a review by Arpino and colleagues [25], which showed that cesarean delivery did not decrease the incidence of cranial ultrasound abnormalities. Of note, however, 77% of the infants in this study were older than 32 weeks of gestation, and white matter injury was the most common abnormality noted in this population.

The Neonatal Brain Hemorrhage Study was a longitudinal cohort study of 1105 infants older than 26 weeks of gestation and with a birth weight of 501 to 2000 g [26]. A standardized protocol for cranial ultrasound screening was used in this study. In addition, these investigators prospectively and systematically collected data defining maternal and neonatal conditions that may affect the primary outcome. In this study, delivery mode was not associated with an increased risk for IVH, Periventricular leukomalacia (PVL), disabling CP or death (Table 1) [26].

Baud and colleagues [27] evaluated pregnancy and neonatal outcomes based on indication for delivery. They stratified infants into groups based on the indication for cesarean section and then evaluated risks for IVH, PVL, and respiratory distress syndrome (RDS). By univariate analysis, cesarean section performed before the onset of labor was associated with a decreased incidence of PVL; however, after adjusting for intrauterine

Table 1
Unadjusted and adjusted odds ratios of labor-delivery status on adverse outcomes

	GM/IVH		PEL/VE		Neonatal death		DCP	
	OR	95% CI	OR	95% CI	OR	95% CI	OR	95% CI
Active labor versus no active labor								
Unadjusted	1.3	0.9–2.0	1.6	0.9–2.6	1.6[a]	1.0–2.8[a]	1.4	0.8–2.5
Adjusted	1.3	0.8–2.1	2.3[a]	1.2–4.5[a]	1.8	0.8–4.0	1.6	0.7–3.7
Vaginal versus cesarean delivery								
Unadjusted	1.0	0.7–1.5	0.9	0.6–1.4	1.0	0.6–1.6	0.9	0.5–1.5
Adjusted	1.0	0.6–1.5	1.0	0.6–1.7	1.3	0.6–2.5	0.9	0.5–1.9

Multivariate model included simultaneous adjustment for labor status or delivery mode, birth weight, GA, multiple gestation, preeclampsia, chorioamnionitis, and placenta abruptio.

Abbreviations: DCP, disabling cerebral palsy; GM, germinal matrix; IVH, intraventricular hemorrhage; PEL, parenchymal echolucencies/echodensities; VE, ventricular enlargement.

[a] Statistically significant OR at the alpha = 0.05 level.

Data from Qiu H, Paneth N, Lorenz JM, et al. Labor and delivery factors in brain damage, disabling cerebral palsy, and neonatal death in low birth weight infants. Am J Obstet Gynecol 2003;189:1148.

growth retardation (IUGR) status and preeclampsia, this difference was no longer statistically significant. Among the subset of infants with intrauterine infection, those delivered by cesarean section had a lower risk for PVL.

The presence of "labor" likely has significance beyond the external force exerted on the fetal head. Infants delivered by elective cesarean section may represent a different patient population with different risk profiles for NDI compared with those who present in active labor. Wadhawan and colleagues [16] performed a retrospective cohort analysis of 1273 ELBW infants weighing less than 1000 g in the National Institute of Child Health and Development (NICHD) Neonatal Research Network who were delivered by cesarean section to determine the impact of active labor on neurodevelopmental outcome at 18 months of adjusted age in this population. They found no significant difference in severe IVH, PVL, or NDI at 18 months of adjusted age in ELBW infants born by cesarean section with or without labor. By univariate analysis, infants born by cesarean section with labor were more likely to have severe IVH, PVL, and NDI; however, after adjusting for potential confounders, including pregnancy-induced hypertension (PIH), GA, and antenatal steroids, there were no significant differences between groups.

Some have suggested that the benefit of cesarean delivery may differ in different GA groups. Malloy and colleagues [1] evaluated neonatal morbidity and mortality in a cohort of 1765 low birth weight infants. IVH was less common in infants delivered by cesarean section; however, this difference was only statistically significantly different in the 1251- to 1500-g subgroup. There was a high mortality rate in the first 24 hours in this historical cohort born between 1987 and 1988, and it was unclear if these findings would be similar in a more contemporary cohort with improved overall survival rates. In a small series of 95 preterm infants, those with a GA greater than 29 weeks and delivered by cesarean section had a lower risk for IVH [28]. Similarly, Deulofeut and colleagues [29] evaluated the short-term outcome and risk for IVH and PVL among a population of 397 infants weighing less than 1251 g. They found that in the subgroup of infants weighing less than 750 g, those delivered vaginally were more likely to have severe IVH compared with those born by cesarean delivery (41% versus 22%).

Vohr and colleagues [8] evaluated the neurodevelopmental outcome of a large cohort of ELBW infants. Mode of delivery by cesarean section was not a predictor of Mental Development Index (MDI) less than 70, Psychomotor Developmental Index (PDI) less than 70, CP, or NDI. Even among the most critically ill ELBW survivors, mode of delivery has not been shown to be a predictor of neurologic outcome [30].

In an analysis of the neurodevelopmental outcome of ELBW infants with severe IVH grade 3 to 4 and posthemorrhagic hydrocephalus, those with grade 3 to 4 IVH and a shunt were more likely to have been delivered vaginally compared with those with no IVH and no shunt [11]. Infants with grade 3 to 4 IVH with and without shunts were more likely to have abnormal neurodevelopmental performance and CP at 18 to 22 months. These data highlight the negative impact of severe IVH on long-term neurodevelopmental outcome.

Improvements in obstetric and neonatal management of the preterm infant have contributed to improved neurodevelopmental outcomes in preterm infants. Nonetheless, caution is recommended in interpretation of data evaluating the impact of mode of delivery on neurologic outcome in the preterm population because of the confounding effect of the associated obstetric complication that is resulting in preterm delivery.

Among vertex-presenting preterm survivors, neonatal morbidity and neurodevelopmental outcome do not seem to be affected by mode of delivery. The American College of Obstetricians and Gynecologists (ACOG) recommends expectant management of the preterm infant and delivery by cesarean delivery only for obstetric indications [31].

Multiple gestation pregnancies

Multiple gestation pregnancies are more likely to be complicated by fetal malpresentation of at least one infant. At present, there are no systematic reviews of neurologic outcome in multiple gestation pregnancies based on mode of delivery. Recommended mode of delivery in multiple gestation pregnancies focuses on obstetric management to minimize the risk for head entrapment, cord prolapse, and birth depression. Each of these complications has been associated with an adverse neurologic outcome [7]. In addition to the presentation of the fetuses, careful assessment of birth weight, growth discordance, and estimated GA should be considered in the decision-making process. If both fetuses are vertex, vaginal delivery is the preferred route of delivery. In contrast, if the presenting fetus is breech, cesarean delivery is usually recommended. If the presenting twin is breech and the second twin is vertex, cesarean delivery is recommended to avoid the risk for "locked" twins when the chins of the infants become locked during the descent process [32]. The recommended delivery mode is unclear when the first twin is vertex and the second twin is breech [33–35] A multicenter randomized controlled trial to evaluate the outcome of twin pregnancy when the presenting twin is vertex and the second twin is in a nonvertex position is ongoing. Researchers are awaiting the results of this important clinical trial.

Cerebral palsy and mode of delivery

CP is a nonprogressive chronic disorder of movement and posture [7,36]. Prematurity is a significant risk factor for development of CP; however, in most cases, the etiology is unknown. The general lack of understanding of the underlying causes of CP has made it difficult to develop effective prevention strategies. Complications during the peripartum period have been associated with approximately 6% of cases of CP in the term population [36,37].

Many investigators believe that the link between CP and perinatal asphyxia has been overestimated, however (Fig. 2) [36,38–40].

Electronic fetal monitoring (EFM) of the fetus during labor was designed to detect alterations in the fetal heart rate tracing that may be indicative of altered perfusion. Initially, perinatologists had hoped that this technology would improve pregnancy and neonatal outcomes; however, several analyses have shown that use of EFM has not been associated with decreased rates of CP, frequency of low Apgar scores, neonatal intensive care unit (NICU) admissions, or death [41–44]. In addition, use of EFM was associated with a 40% increase in cesarean deliveries [43]. EFM has a low specificity for identifying children who are likely to develop CP. The false-positive rate has been estimated at 99.8% [40]. Among infants with abnormalities on EFM during the intrapartum period, the mode of delivery was not associated with the risk for development of CP. There were similar rates of CP among infants delivered by cesarean delivery and vaginally. Similar disappointing results have been reported for the use of fetal pulse oximetry as a predictor of outcome.

Some have speculated that mode of delivery is related to risk for CP. Krebs and Langhoff-Roos [45] performed a case-control study to evaluate the relation between breech presentation at term and risk for CP. Breech presentation was slightly more common in infants with CP; however, after adjustment for gestational and small for gestational age (SGA) status, the differences were no longer significant. Mode of delivery was not associated with an increased risk for CP. A significant percentage of children who develop CP have a history of perinatal depression that may have prompted cesarean delivery; however, this information does not establish a causal relation between mode of delivery and CP. In this instance, cesarean delivery is simply an indicator of a high-risk population with other risk factors.

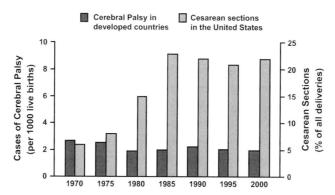

Fig. 2. Prevalence of CP and the rate of cesarean delivery in developed countries. Pooled data are from Australia, Canada, Denmark, England, Ireland, Norway, Scotland, Sweden, and the United States. (*From* Nelson KB. Can we prevent cerebral palsy? N Engl J Med 2003;139: 1768; with permission. Copyright © 2003, Massachusetts Medical Society.)

Apgar scores are used to assess the overall physiologic stability of a newborn immediately after birth. Historically, attempts were made to find an association between low Apgar scores and neurologic outcome. This association has not been well supported, particularly for the 1- and 5-minute Apgar scores. The ACOG has issued guidelines for the determination of perinatal asphyxia [46]. Low Apgar scores alone do not represent sufficient evidence for a perinatal cause of neurologic injury. Additional perinatal factors must be present to diagnose asphyxia, including 10-minute Apgar scores of 0 to 3, early neonatal seizures, and prolonged hypotonia [47].

Despite the exponential increase in the elective cesarean delivery rate, the incidence of CP has remained relatively constant. Therefore, indirectly, one can infer that obstetric complications and mode of delivery are not the only determinants of this adverse neurologic outcome.

Breech presentation and mode of delivery

Approximately 3% to 4% of infants at term and up to 30% of VLBW infants have breech presentation at delivery [37,48,49]. Complications of breech delivery associated with neurologic compromise include an increased risk for cord prolapse, head entrapment, and birth trauma [32,50]. The optimum mode of delivery for the term and preterm breech-presenting infant has been actively debated. Evidence-based recommendations have been derived from multiple well-designed clinical trials evaluating mortality and short-term and long-term morbidity, including neurodevelopmental outcome.

Term infants and breech presentation

Early observational studies suggested an improved outcome and decreased mortality if term breech infants were delivered by means of cesarean section [51–56].

Gilbert and colleagues [51] performed a large population-based retrospective analysis of more than 3 million births in California between 1991 and 1998 to evaluate pregnancy outcomes associated with vaginal breech delivery in term infants. In this study, vaginal breech delivery was associated with a significantly increased risk for neonatal mortality (OR = 9.2, 95% CI: 3.3–25.6) and morbidity, including asphyxia, brachial plexus injury, and birth trauma for a nulliparous woman when compared with the outcome of breech delivery by cesarean delivery for a nulliparous woman [51]. Among women with a history of at least one prior vaginal delivery, there was no difference in mortality based on mode of delivery; however, the risk for serious neonatal morbidity, including asphyxia, brachial plexus injury, and birth trauma, were all significantly higher in the vaginal delivery group. There was a high incidence of brachial plexus injury in vaginal breech deliveries (0.9%) compared with cephalic vaginal deliveries (0.1%) and breech cesarean deliveries (<0.1%).

In a large population-based retrospective analysis of pregnancy outcomes among 15,818 term infants in breech position, researchers again found a significantly decreased mortality rate among those delivered by means of cesarean section. Infants delivered vaginally were more likely to have adverse neurologic outcome, including seizures and birth trauma [52]. Kiely [53] reported similar results among a cohort of 17,587 breech deliveries in New York City.

A Swedish study also reported that all adverse outcomes occurred more frequently in the planned vaginal delivery group compared with those delivered by elective cesarean section [49]. A significant number of infants in the vaginal delivery group also had evidence of hypoxic ischemic encephalopathy and brachial plexus injury.

The Term Breech Trial was a pivotal study. A total of 2088 women with breech-presenting fetuses were randomized to a planned vaginal delivery or a planned cesarean section. There were no differences in maternal morbidity or mortality; however, neonatal morbidity and mortality were significantly decreased in infants delivered by cesarean section [57]. Seventy-nine percent of the original cohort had a neurodevelopmental assessment at 2 years of age [58]. This follow-up study used the Ages and Stages Questionnaire (ASQ) to survey developmental skills based on parent report. Those infants with an abnormal score had a neurologic examination performed. The risk for death or neurodevelopmental delay was similar between those delivered by planned cesarean birth (3.1%) and those delivered by planned vaginal birth (2.8%); (relative risk [RR] = 1.09, 95% CI: 0.52–2.30; P = .85). Even though this is important developmental follow-up data, these results should be reviewed with caution because there are several methodologic concerns that question the generalizability of these findings. All study subjects did not have a standardized neurologic examination, which could have resulted in an underestimate of impairment. The ASQ is based on parent report, which many do not consider a reliable source for more subtle neurologic abnormalities. Most important, the investigators who conducted this trial acknowledge that the follow-up component of this study was only powered to detect large differences between the two groups. Despite these study limitations, we should not minimize the importance of this clinical trial because it provides a baseline risk for death or long-term NDI in the term breech population and shows us that there were no large differences in long-term NDI between the term breech infants delivered vaginally or by means of cesarean delivery [58].

Furthermore, Danielian and colleagues [59] and Gravenhorst and colleagues [60] have reported neurodevelopmental outcome at 4 to 5 years of age in term breech infants and found no difference in neurologic disability rates based on mode of delivery.

In contrast, Molkenboer and colleagues [61] from The Netherlands evaluated neurodevelopmental outcome data at 2 years but stratified by birth weight. They evaluated all patients at their center who presented in breech presentation at term who were not participants in the Term Breech Trial. Among the 203 infants studied, they found that those infants with birth weight greater than 3500 g were more likely to have abnormal development at 2 years of age, based on responses to the ASQ. The same methodologic concerns previously mentioned about the Term Breech Trial also apply to interpretation of this study because of the inadequate sample size to detect smaller differences between the groups.

After the long-term neurodevelopmental outcome data from the International Term Breech Trial found no difference in neurologic outcome at 2 years of age, some investigators began to question the recommendation for elective cesarean delivery of term breech infants [62]. Nevertheless, one must question whether this is the appropriate benchmark to evaluate the impact of mode of delivery on neurologic outcome in this population. The lack of improvement in long-term neurodevelopmental outcome does not negate the clear improvement in mortality and early morbidity rates, including brachial plexus injury and birth trauma. In addition, we must remember that even though the Term Breech Trial is the largest published study of neurodevelopmental outcome of this subset of infants, the investigators who conducted this trial clearly acknowledge that this study was not adequately powered to detect more modest yet clinically significant differences in neurodevelopmental outcome between the two groups.

The 2006 ACOG consensus opinion provides guidelines for delivery of the breech term infant [35]. The ACOG states that elective cesarean section is the preferred route of delivery in most situations because of the decreased number of clinicians with adequate clinical expertise to perform a vaginal breech delivery. Given that the long-term outcome data showed no difference in neurodevelopmental outcome at 2 years, however, vaginal breech delivery is considered a reasonable option for select patients. Mothers must be appropriately counseled on risks associated with attempting vaginal breech delivery. Patients should be carefully selected to avoid unnecessary morbidity.

Preterm and breech presentation

Obstetricians have become hypervigilant in the care and management of the preterm infant in an effort to improve neurologic outcome in this high-risk group of patients. In general, preterm infants are at higher risk for neurologic injury secondary to the limited ability of the preterm brain to autoregulate cerebral perfusion during periods of hypoxia and asphyxia [7,32,50]. The preterm breech infant being delivered vaginally through a partially dilated cervix is also at risk for head entrapment.

Unlike the term breech population, there are no randomized controlled trials to evaluate the impact of mode of delivery on neurodevelopmental outcome in the preterm breech population. Available data from several retrospective reviews have reported variable findings. Birth weight seems to modify the risk analysis for adverse neurologic outcome in the preterm breech population.

In a single-center study of 1009 VLBW infants (<1500 g) in breech presentation, those delivered by cesarean section had lower perinatal mortality and decreased neonatal morbidity [50]. After adjusting for birth weight, infants weighing 750 to 999 g had a statistically significantly improved survival rate based on mode of delivery (66% versus 23.3%; $P<.001$). Similarly, preterm breech infants delivered vaginally had a higher incidence of grade 3 or 4 IVH (18.8% versus 3.5%; $P<.001$), were more likely to have 5-minute Apgar scores less than 4 (11.6% versus 1.2%; $P<.001$), and had a higher incidence of necrotizing enterocolitis (NEC) when compared with those delivered by means of cesarean delivery. Muhuri and colleagues [56] also reported improved short-term morbidity among VLBW infants delivered by cesarean section.

Main and colleagues [63] performed an analysis of preterm infants weighing less than 1500 g. They noted a decreased mortality rate but no difference in neonatal neurologic morbidity, including incidence of IVH.

Various analyses have reported that the mode of delivery is not associated with increased neonatal mortality in the VLBW population after controlling for obstetric risk factors, birth weight, and GA [1,64–67]. Among breech-presenting VLBW infants, the ideal mode of delivery has been questioned. Although somewhat limited, the available data suggest that breech-presenting VLBW infants should be delivered by cesarean section. Infants weighing less than 1500 g seem to have the most consistent advantage of cesarean delivery.

Brachial plexus and spinal cord injury and mode of delivery

Brachial plexus injury has a reported occurrence rate of 0.05% to 0.25% [68,69]. Although rare, permanent injury to the brachial plexus represents significant morbidity with long-term implications on motor functioning. In addition, affected infants are more likely to have a history of birth asphyxia, which may also have an impact on long-term neurologic outcome [68]. The risk for brachial plexus injury varies with fetal presentation and mode of delivery (Fig. 3).

Brachial plexus injury occurs almost exclusively in term infants and is primarily believed to be a result of traumatic injury to the nerve roots of the brachial plexus during the delivery process. These nerve roots are stretched and injured during extreme lateral traction, which is exerted by the shoulder when delivering the head with breech presentation or by the head when delivering the shoulder in cephalic presentation [7]. There are several case reports of brachial plexus injury in deliveries with no apparent trauma or traction or involving the posterior arm, however [70–73]. This has led some investigators to believe that some cases are secondary to an intrauterine event.

Risk factors for brachial plexus injury include fetal macrosomia greater than 4500 g, macrocephaly, malpresentation, and shoulder dystocia

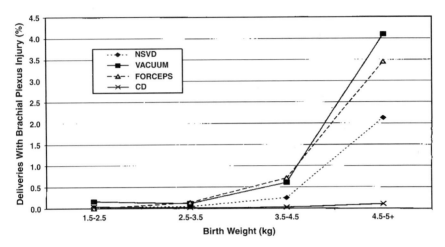

Fig. 3. Frequency of brachial plexus injury stratified by birth weight and displayed as mode of delivery. CD, cesarean delivery; NSVD, normal spontaneous vaginal delivery. (*From* Gilbert WM, Nesbitt TS, Danielsen B. Associated factors in 1611 cases of brachial plexus injury. Obstet Gynecol 1999;83:537; with permission).

[7,51,68,69]. Gordon and colleagues [74] reported that among infants with brachial plexus injury, 56% had an abnormal presentation (14% breech and 42% occiput posterior or occiput transverse). Maternal obesity seems to increase the risk for brachial plexus injury independently in deliveries complicated by shoulder dystocia [69,75].

In a large, retrospective, population-based cohort study of term infants in the state of California, the risk for brachial plexus injury was ninefold higher in vaginal breech deliveries (0.9%) compared with cephalic vaginal deliveries (0.1%) or breech cesarean delivery (<0.1%). Cesarean delivery of the breech fetus was protective against brachial plexus injury [51]. Similar to previous reports, in this cohort, the RR of brachial plexus injury increased with increasing birth weight, gestational diabetes, and operative vaginal delivery.

Clinical presentation

There is significant variability in the severity of neurologic impairment associated with brachial plexus injury, ranging from transient weakness to complete paralysis. The clinical presentation correlates to the severity of the injury (Table 2). The most common form of brachial plexus injury is neurapraxia, which occurs when there is injury to the nerve sheath with associated hemorrhage and edema but the axons are intact. Axonal dysfunction occurs as a result of compression from the swelling in the surrounding tissues. Most of these patients have complete recovery. In contrast, a positive outcome is less likely when the axons or nerve roots are severed or ruptured [7].

Table 2
Relation of pathologic findings to likelihood of spontaneous recovery in brachial plexus injury

Severity of lesion	Nerve sheath	Axons	Roots	Likelihood of spontaneous recovery
Mild	Injured	Intact	Intact	Good
Moderate	Intact	Severed	Intact	Fair
Severe	Severed	Severed	Intact	Poor
Severe	Intact	Intact	Severed	Poor

Data from Volpe JJ. Neurology of the newborn. 4th edition. Philadelphia: WB Saunders; 2001. p. 826.

Erb's palsy is caused by injury to the nerve roots C5 to C6 as they join to form the upper trunk of the brachial plexus (Erb's point). Fifty percent of cases also involve the C7 root. Approximately 5% of affected patients have ipsilateral diaphragmatic paralysis also. Injury to this proximal nerve root results in the limb being held in the classic "waiter's tip" position with the arm adducted, internally rotated, and pronated. On physical examination, the biceps reflex (C5, C6) may be absent. The infant has an asymmetric Moro reflex, and there is often minimal or no response of the affected side. Affected infants typically have a normal grasp reflex because innervation to finger flexors is preserved (Table 3) [7].

Klumpke's palsy is caused by injury to the point at which C8 to T1 joins to form the lower trunk of the brachial plexus. Affected infants have weakness in the distal upper extremity.

Patients who have complete brachial plexus injury have evidence of weakness in the upper and lower brachial plexus nerve roots. Approximately one third of affected infants also have sympathetic dysfunction and Horner's syndrome with associated ptosis, miosis, and anhidrosis. Affected infants have the findings described for Erb's palsy; in addition, the grasp reflex is absent.

There are limited data on the risk for recurrent brachial plexus injury in subsequent pregnancies [74,76]. Several small case series reports have been

Table 3
Major pattern of weakness with brachial plexus injury

Area of weakness	Cord segment involved	Muscle group involved	Resulting position
Shoulder abduction	C5	Deltoid	Adducted
Shoulder external rotation	C5	Spinati	Internally rotated
Elbow flexion	C5, C6	Biceps and Brachioradialis	Extended
Supination	C5, C6	Biceps, Supinator	Pronated
Wrist extension	C6, C7		Flexed
Finger extension	C6, C7		Flexed
Diaphragmatic descent	C4, C5		Elevated hemidiaphragm

Data from Volpe JJ. Neurology of the newborn. 4th edition. Philadelphia: WB Saunders; 2001. p. 827.

published suggesting that these women are at somewhat higher risk for injury in subsequent pregnancies. In particular, those with a history of permanent brachial plexus injury seem more likely to have a recurrent brachial plexus injury in subsequent pregnancies. Some believe that it is reasonable to offer elective cesarean delivery to women with a child with permanent brachial plexus injury [68,74,76].

Prognosis

Historically, it was reported that most patients have complete recovery. In a recent review by Hoeksma and colleagues [77], however, they reported that only 66% of patients have complete recovery. Prognosis correlated directly with the severity of the injury. Recovery of function within 2 to 4 weeks is a favorable prognostic sign. Most infants with brachial plexus injury have resolution of symptoms by 4 months of age, and up to 92% are normal by 12 months of age [7,51,78]. Microsurgical techniques for brachial plexus reconstruction are being performed in some centers in children with delayed return of function [79,80].

Spinal cord injury

Spinal cord injury is a rare but potentially devastating event that is usually associated with birth trauma causing excessive traction or torsion on the spinal cord. A significant percentage of affected infants have malpresentation; however, cases of infants in cephalic presentation have also been described. Cord injury occurs secondary to traction on the trunk during breech delivery, hyperextension of the head in vaginal breech delivery, or traction during shoulder dystocia [7].

There are two primary sections of the spinal cord that are typically involved. Lower cervical or upper thoracic lesions are more common in breech deliveries. Middle upper cervical lesions are more common in cephalic presentations [7]. In cases in which the injury seems to occur in utero, it is likely secondary to subluxation of the upper cervical vertebrae.

Affected infants often have depressed or absent respiratory effort; muscle weakness, hypotonia, and abdominal breathing are common. These infants are areflexic and may have evidence of sympathetic dysfunction. In addition to the motor impairment, affected infants have a high mortality rate in early childhood. Although not completely preventable, some cases of spinal cord injury can be avoided by performing cesarean delivery on obviously at-risk patients.

References

[1] Malloy MH, Onstad L, Wright E, NICHD Neonatal Research Network. The effect of cesarean delivery on birth outcome in very low birth weight infants. Obstet Gynecol 1991;77(4): 498–503.

[2] Shankaran S, Fanaroff AA, Wright LL, et al. Risk factors for early death among extremely low-birth-weight infants. Am J Obstet Gynecol 2002;186(4):796–802.

[3] Haywood JL, Morse SB, Goldenberg RL, et al. Estimation of outcome and restriction of interventions in neonates. Pediatrics 1998;102:e6.

[4] Haywood JL, Goldenberg RL, Bronstein J, et al. Comparison of perceived and actual rates of survival and freedom from handicap in premature infants. Am J Obstet Gynecol 1994;171: 432–9.

[5] Lee HC, Gould JB. Survival advantage associated with cesarean delivery in very low birth weight vertex neonates. Obstet Gynecol 2006;107:97–105.

[6] Jonas HA, Lumley JM. The effect of mode of delivery on neonatal mortality in very low birthweight infants born in Victoria, Australia: caesarean section is associated with increased survival in breech-presenting, but not vertex-presenting, infants. Paediatr Perinat Epidemiol 1997;11:181–99.

[7] Volpe JJ. Neurology of the newborn. 4th edition. Philadelphia: WB Saunders; 2001.

[8] Vohr BR, Wright LL, Dusick AM, et al. Neurodevelopmental and functional outcomes of extremely low birth weight infants in the National Institute of Child Health and Human Development Neonatal Research Network, 1993–1994. Pediatrics 2000;105(6):1216–26.

[9] Hintz SR, Kendrick DE, Vohr BR, et al. Changes in neurodevelopmental outcomes at 18–22 months' corrected age among infants of less than 25 weeks' gestational age born 1993–1999. Pediatrics 2005;115(6):1645–51.

[10] Wilson-Costello D, Friedman H, Minich N, et al. Improved survival rates with increased neurodevelopmental disability for extremely low birth weight infants in the 1990s. Pediatrics 2005;115:997–1003.

[11] Adams-Chapman I, Hansen NI, Higgin R, et al. NICHD Neonatal Research Network. Neurodevelopmental outcome of ELBW infants with posthemorrhagic hydrocephalus requiring shunt insertion. Pediatrics 2008;121(5):e1167–77.

[12] Ment LR, Allan WC, Makuch RW, et al. Grade 3 to 4 intraventricular hemorrhage and Bayley scores predict outcome. Pediatrics 2005;116:1597–8.

[13] Ment LR, Vohr B, Allan W, et al. Outcome of children in the indomethacin intraventricular hemorrhage prevention trial. Pediatrics 2000;105:485–91.

[14] Ment LR, Oh W, Philip AG, et al. Risk factors for early intraventricular hemorrhage in low birth weight infants. J Pediatr 1992;121(5):776–83.

[15] Anderson P, Doyle LW, Victorian Infant Collaborative Study Group. Neurobehavioral outcomes of school-age children born extremely low birth weight or very preterm in the 1990's. JAMA 2003;289:3264–72.

[16] Wadhawan R, Bohr BR, Fanaroff AA, et al. Does labor influence neonatal and neurodevelopmental outcomes of extremely low birth weight infants who are born by cesarean delivery? Am J Obstet Gynecol 2003;189:501–6.

[17] Welch RA, Bottoms SF. Reconsideration of head compression and intraventricular hemorrhage in the vertex, very low birth weight fetus. Obstet Gynecol 1986;68(1):29.

[18] Bejar R, Curbelo V, Coen R, et al. Large intraventricular hemorrhage (IVH) and labor in infants greater than or equal to 1000 g. Pediatr Res 1981;15:649.

[19] Bishop EH, Isreal SL, Criscoe CC. Obstetric influences on the premature infant's first year of development. A report from the Collaborative Study of Cerebral Palsy. Obstet Gynecol 1965;25:628.

[20] Bowes WA. Delivery of the very low birth weight infant. Clin Perinatol 1981;8:183.

[21] Tejani N, Verma U, Hameed C, et al. Method and route of delivery in the low birth weight vertex presentation correlated with early periventricular/intraventricular hemorrhage. Obstet Gynecol 1987;69:1–4.

[22] Paul DA, Sciscione A, Leef KH, et al. Caesarean delivery and outcome in very low birth-weight infants. Aust N Z J Obstet Gynaecol 2002;42:41–5.

[23] Newton ER, Haering WA, Kennedy JL, et al. Effect of mode of delivery on morbidity and mortality of infants at early gestational age. Obstet Gynecol 1986;67:507–11.

[24] Vergani P, Locatelli A, Doria V, et al. Intraventricular hemorrhage and periventricular leukomalacia in preterm infants. Obstet Gynecol 2004;104:225–31.

[25] Arpino C, Brescianini S, Ticconi C, et al. Does cesarean section prevent mortality and cerebral ultrasound abnormalities in preterm newborns? J Matern Fetal Med 2007;20(2):151–9.

[26] Qiu H, Paneth N, Lorenz JM, et al. Labor and delivery factors in brain damage, disabling cerebral palsy, and neonatal death in low birth weight infants. Am J Obstet Gynecol 2003; 189:1143–9.

[27] Baud O, Zupan V, Lacaze-Masmonteil T, et al. The relationships between antenatal management, the cause of delivery and neonatal outcome in a large cohort of very preterm singleton infants. Br J Obstet Gynaecol 2000;107:877–84.

[28] Dolfin T, Skidmore MB, Fong KW, et al. Perinatal factors that influence the incidence of subependymal and intraventricular hemorrhage in low birthweight infants. Am J Perinatol 1984;1(2):107–13.

[29] Deulofeut R, Sola A, Lee B, et al. The impact of vaginal delivery in premature infants weighing less than 1,251 grams. Obstet Gynecol 2005;105(3):525–31.

[30] Shankaran S, Johnson Y, Langer JC, et al. Outcome of extremely low birth weight infants at highest risk: gestational age < or = 24 weeks, birth weight < or = 750 g, and 1 minute Apgar < or = 3. Am J Obstet Gynecol 2004;19(4):1084–91.

[31] Grant A, Glazener CMA. Elective caesarean section versus expectant management for delivery of the small baby. Systematic review. Cochrane Pregnancy and Childbirth Group. Cochrane Database Syst Rev 2007;4.

[32] Yamamura Y, Ramin KD, Ramin SM. Trial of vaginal breech delivery: current role. Clin Obstet Gynecol 2007;50(2):526–36.

[33] Sibony O, Touitou S, Luton D, et al. Modes of delivery of first and second twins as a function of their presentation. Eur J Obstet Gynecol Reprod Biol 2006;126(2):180–5.

[34] Yang Q, Wen SW, Chen Y, et al. Neonatal death and morbidity in vertex-non-vertex second twin according to mode of delivery and birth weight. Am J Obstet Gynecol 2005;192(3): 840–7.

[35] American College of Obstetricians and Gynecologists. Mode of term singleton breech delivery. ACOG Committee opinion number 340. Washington, DC: American College of Obstetricians and Gynecologists; 2006.

[36] Nelson KB, Grether JK. Potentially asphyxiating conditions and spastic cerebral palsy in infants of normal birth weight. Am J Obstet Gynecol 1998;179:507–13.

[37] Gary Cunningham F. Williams' obstetrics. 22nd edition. New York: McGraw Hill Publishing; 2005.

[38] American College of Obstetricians and Gynecologists Task Force on Neonatal Encephalopathy and Cerebral Palsy, American College of Obstetricians and Gynecologists, American Academy of Pediatrics. Neonatal encephalopathy and cerebral palsy: defining the pathogenesis and pathophysiology. Washington, DC: American College of Obstetricians and Gynecologists; 2003.

[39] Tyson JE, Gilstrap LC. Hope for perinatal prevention of cerebral palsy. JAMA 2003;290: 2730–2.

[40] Nelson KB. Can we prevent cerebral palsy? N Engl J Med 2003;139(18):1765–9.

[41] Grant A, O'Brien N, Joy MT, et al. Cerebral palsy among children born during the Dublin randomised trial of intrapartum monitoring. Lancet 1989;2:1233–6.

[42] Shy KK, Luthy DA, Bennett FC, et al. Effects of electronic fetal heart rate monitoring, as compared with periodic auscultation, on the neurologic development of premature infants. N Engl J Med 1990;322:588–93.

[43] Thacker SB, Stroup D, Chang M. Continuous electronic heart rate monitoring for fetal assessment during labor. Cochrane Database Syst Rev 2001;(2):CD000063.

[44] Alfirevic Z, Devane D, Gyte GML. Continuous cardiotocography (CTG) as a form of electronic fetal monitoring (EFM) for fetal assessment during labor. Cochrane Database Syst Rev 2008;1:CD006066.

[45] Krebs L, Langhoff-Roos J. The relation of breech presentation at term to epilepsy in childhood. Eur J Obstet Gynecol Reprod Biol 2006;127:26–8, NO.

[46] American College of Obstetricians and Gynecologists. Inappropriate use of the term fetal distress and asphyxia. Committee opinion number 326. Obstet Gynecol 2005;106(6):1469–70.

[47] Ellenberg JH, Nelson KB. Cluster of perinatal events identifying infants at high risk for death or disability. J Pediatr 1988;113:546.

[48] Hickok DE, Gordon DC, Milberg JA, et al. The frequency of breech presentation by gestational age at birth: a large population-based study. Am J Obstet Gynecol 1992;166:851–6.

[49] Herbst A, Thorngren-Jerneck K. Mode of delivery in breech presentation at term: increased neonatal morbidity with vaginal delivery. Acta Obstet Gynecol Scand 2001;80:731–7.

[50] Görbe E, Chasen S, Harmath A, et al. Very-low birthweight infants: short term outcome by method of delivery. J Matern Fetal Med 1997;155–8.

[51] Gilbert WM, Hicks SM, Boe NM, et al. Vaginal versus cesarean delivery for breech presentation in California: a population-based study. Obstet Gynecol 2003;102:911–7.

[52] Roman J, Bakos O, Cnattingius S. Pregnancy outcomes by mode of delivery among term breech births: Swedish experience 1987–1993. Obstet Gynecol 1998;92(6):945–50.

[53] Kiely JL. Mode of delivery and neonatal death in 17,587 infants presenting by breech. Br J Obstet Gynaecol 1991;898–904.

[54] Villar J, Carroli G, Zavaleta N, et al, World Health Organization 2005 Global Survey on Maternal and Perinatal Health Research Group. Maternal and neonatal individual risks and benefits associated with caesarean delivery: multicentre prospective study. BMJ 2007; 335:1025.

[55] Villar J, Valladares E, Wojdyla D, et al. Caesarean delivery rates and pregnancy outcomes: the 2005 WHO Global Survey on Maternal and Perinatal Health in Latin America. Lancet 2006;367:1819–29.

[56] Muhuri PK, MacDorman MF, Menacker F. Method of delivery and neonatal mortality among very low-birth-weight infants in the United States. Matern Child Health J 2006;10: 47–53.

[57] Hannah ME, Hannah WJ, Hewson SA, et al. Planned caesarean section versus planned vaginal birth for breech presentation at term: a randomized multicentre trial. Lancet 2000;356: 1375–83.

[58] Whyte H, Hannah ME, Saigal S, et al. Outcomes of children at 2 years after planned cesarean birth versus planned vaginal birth for breech presentation at term: the International Randomized Term Breech Trial. Am J Obstet Gynecol 2004;191:864–71.

[59] Danielian PJ, Wang J, Hall MH. Long term outcome by mode of delivery of fetuses in breech presentation at term: population based follow up. BMJ 1996;312:1451–3.

[60] Gravenhorst JB, Veen S, Verloove-Vanhorick SP, et al. Breech delivery in very preterm and very low birthweight infants in the Netherlands. Br J Obstet Gynaecol 1993;100:411–5.

[61] Molkenboer JF, Roumen FJ, Smits LJ, et al. Birth weight and neurodevelopmental outcome of children at 2 years of age after planned vaginal delivery for breech presentation at term. Am J Obstet Gynecol 2006;194:624–9.

[62] Sanchez-Ramos L, Wells TL, Adair CD, et al. Route of breech delivery and maternal and neonatal outcomes. Int J Gynaecol Obstet 2001;73:7–14.

[63] Main DM, Main EK, Maurer MM. Cesarean section versus vaginal delivery for the breech fetus weighing less than 1,500 grams. Am J Obstet Gynecol 1983;146(5):580–4.

[64] Jonas HA, Khalid N, Schwartz SM. The relationship between caesarean section and neonatal mortality in very-low-birth-weight infants born in Washington State, USA. Paediatr Perinat Epidemiol 1999;13:170–89.

[65] Kitchen W, Ford GW, Doyle LW, et al. Cesarean section or vaginal delivery at 24 to 28 weeks gestation: comparison of survival and neonatal and two-year morbidity. Obstet Gynecol 1985;66:149–57.

[66] Herschel M, Kennedy JL Jr, Kayne HL, et al. Survival of infants born at 24 to 28 weeks gestation. Obstet Gynecol 1982;60(2):154–8.

[67] Worthington D, Davis LE, Graug JP, et al. Factors influencing survival and morbidity with very-low-birth-weight delivery. Obstet Gynecol 1983;63:550.

[68] Gilbert WM, Nesbitt TS, Danielsen B. Associated factors in 1611 cases of brachial plexus injury. Obstet Gynecol 1999;83:536–40.

[69] Mehta SH, Blackwell SC, Jujold E, et al. What factors are associated with neonatal injury following shoulder dystocia? J Perinatol 2006;26:85–8.

[70] Jennett RJ, Tarby TJ. Brachial plexus palsy: an old problem revisited again. Am J Obstet Gynecol 1997;176:1354–7.

[71] Ouzounian JG, Korst LM, Phelan JP. Permanent Erb palsy: a traction-related injury? Obstet Gynecol 1997;89:139–41.

[72] Lerner HM, Salamon E. Permanent brachial plexus injury following vaginal delivery without physician traction or shoulder dystocia. Am J Obstet Gynecol 2008;e1–2.

[73] Hankins GD, Clark SL. Brachial plexus palsy involving the posterior shoulder at spontaneous vaginal delivery. Am J Perinatol 1995;12:44–5.

[74] Gordon M, Rich H, Deutschberger J, et al. The immediate and long term outcome of obstetric birth trauma. I. Brachial plexus paralysis. Am J Obstet Gynecol 1973;117:51–6.

[75] Cedergren MI. Maternal morbid obesity and the risk of adverse outcome. Obstet Gynecol 2004;103:219–24.

[76] Al-Quattan MM, Al-Kharfy TM. Obstetric brachial plexus injury in subsequent deliveries. Ann Plast Surg 1996;37:545–8.

[77] Hoeksma AF, ter Steeg AM, Nelissen RG, et al. Neurological recovery in obstetrical brachial plexus injuries: an historical cohort study. Dev Med Child Neurol 2004;46:76–83.

[78] Nocon JJ, McKenzie DK, Thomas LJ, et al. Shoulder dystocia: an analysis of risks and obstetric maneuvers. Am J Obstet Gynecol 1993;168:1732–7.

[79] Kirjavainen M, Remes V, Peltonen J, et al. Long-term results of surgery for brachial plexus birth palsy. J Bone Joint Surg Am 2007;89(1):18–26.

[80] Strombeck C, Krumlinde-Sundholm L, Forssberg H. Functional outcome at 5 years in children with obstetrical brachial plexus palsy with and without microsurgical reconstruction. Dev Med Child Neurol 2000;42:148–57.

ELSEVIER
SAUNDERS

CLINICS IN
PERINATOLOGY

Clin Perinatol 35 (2008) 455–462

The Ethical Debate of Maternal Choice and Autonomy in Cesarean Delivery

Helen O. Williams, MD

*Department of Pediatrics, Emory University School of Medicine,
Atlanta, GA 30322, USA*

In recent years there has been much commentary in the obstetric and neonatal literature and in the news media about the rising rates of cesarean births. In particular, attention has been paid to those cesarean sections believed to have been performed without a clear medical or obstetric indication, so-called "cesarean delivery on maternal request" (CDMR). Data from the National Center for Health Statistics show cesarean deliveries in the United States at the highest level ever reported. In 2005, 30.3% of live births in the United States were delivered by cesarean section [1]. Of these cesarean births, 62% were primary or first cesarean birth. Primary cesarean delivery is increasing at a rate parallel to that of total cesarean deliveries [2]. Estimates of the extent of CDMR vary, ranging between 4% and 18% of all cesarean deliveries [3,4].

In 2006, the National Institutes of Health (NIH) convened a consensus conference on CDMR [2]. The panel determined that there is insufficient evidence to compare the benefits and risks of CDMR with planned vaginal delivery. They concluded that the decision to perform CDMR should be individualized and consistent with ethical principles. This article reviews the current ethical debate surrounding CDMR.

Autonomy

The principle of respect for autonomy recognizes the importance of helping patients be as self-determined as possible. It is the principle cited most often as supporting CDMR. Fundamental to respecting autonomy is a commitment to educating patients and ensuring that fully informed consent for treatments occurs. Patients cannot make an autonomous decision unless they are adequately informed and understand the benefits and burdens of

E-mail address: howilli@emory.edu

doi:10.1016/j.clp.2008.03.011
perinatology.theclinics.com

the procedure they are considering. It becomes challenging to obtain informed consent when benefits and risks of a given procedure are not understood clearly; such is the case in CDMR. The recent NIH consensus conference highlighted the paucity of good studies comparing outcomes between planned cesarean deliveries and planned vaginal birth [2].

Autonomy generally grants to patients a negative right, that is to say they have the ability to decline a particular therapy or to not have a treatment forced on them. Patients may not be afforded a positive right of autonomy (ie, patients are not allowed to demand what their physicians consider an unnecessary and potentially harmful therapy). It is unclear in CDMR whether or not patients are asserting a positive right or simply choosing between two modes of delivery that are comparable.

The United States emphasis on autonomy and away from paternalism (physician-directed care) makes some physicians reluctant to advise their patients. Making a recommendation for treatment may be compatible, however, with supporting patients' autonomy and is considered by many ethics scholars as essential to informed consent. Seven elements essential for informed consent are identifiable (Box 1) [5].

Educating patients about cesarean delivery requires physicians to discuss not only the risks and benefits of the procedure but also the potential short- and long-term risks and benefits for the mothers and infants. The limitations of the available evidence also should be shared with patients to help inform their decision. The evidence for and against CDMR is discussed in the following sections.

Beneficence and nonmaleficence

The principle of beneficence recognizes the importance of promoting good or doing what is in the best interest of a patient. A companion principle is that of nonmaleficence, the obligation to avoid harming a patient. The

---

Box 1. Seven elements essential for informed consent

1. Threshold elements (preconditions)
   a. Competence (to understand and decide)
   b. Voluntariness (in deciding)
2. Information elements
   a. Disclosure (of material information)
   b. Recommendation (of a plan)
   c. Understanding (of a and b)
3. Consent elements
   a. Decision (in favor of the plan)
   b. Authorization (of chosen plan)

difficulty with CDMR may lie in balancing the best interests of the pregnant woman, while minimizing potential harms for her and her fetus/newborn.

The primary benefit for mothers cited most often as justifying CDMR is prevention of pelvic floor disorders, including urinary and fecal incontinence and pelvic organ prolapse [4,6–9]. A recent NIH consensus conference found, however, that the evidence supporting CDMR on the grounds of prevention of pelvic floor disorders was weak because only a few randomized controlled trials have addressed this outcome variable. Analysis of women enrolled in one trial, the Term Breech Trial, showed that those women who underwent planned cesarean delivery were at a lower risk for incontinence 3 months post partum [10]. At 2 years post partum, however, the rates of urinary incontinence, although higher in the planned vaginal delivery group, no longer reached statistical significance [11]. Although the Term Breech Trial was a randomized control trial, it was designed to study neonatal, not maternal, outcomes.

In a second study, a large cohort study published in *The New England Journal of Medicine*, the risk for urinary incontinence was found higher among women who had a vaginal delivery than women who had a cesarean delivery [12]. Women who delivered by either method were at greater risk for urinary incontinence than nulliparous women.

Results of the Childbirth and Pelvic Symptoms [13] study compared urinary incontinence between women who delivered vaginally and by cesarean section. Although urinary incontinence was more prevalent in the vaginal cohort than the cesarean cohort, the difference was not statistically significant.

In her review of this topic, Nygaard [14] concluded that vaginal delivery itself is neither always sufficient nor necessary to cause urinary incontinence in most women. Also, cesarean delivery is not sufficient to prevent all urinary incontinence.

From a nonmaleficence perspective, CDMR carries risks for future pregnancies that must be discussed thoroughly with pregnant women [15]. The risk for placental abnormalities, especially placenta previa, increases with the number of prior cesarean deliveries [16]. This risk must be placed in the context of other factors associated with placenta previa, however, such as advancing maternal age and multiparity, which often coexist in women seeking cesarean deliveries. The risks for placenta accreta and hysterectomy also increase as the number of cesarean deliveries increases [15]. Other serious maternal morbidities seen more frequently with increasing cesareans include cystotomy, bowel injury and ileus, ureteral injury, and the need for postoperative ventilation [15]. For these reasons, CDMR should be discouraged in women planning multiple pregnancies and these risks should be with all women expressing an interest in cesarean delivery.

Potential benefits to newborns afforded by cesarean birth include prevention of intracranial hemorrhage, neonatal asphyxia, encephalopathy, birth injury, and reduced neonatal infection [2,17]. A large case-control study showed a greater rate of intracranial hemorrhage in infants delivered by vacuum extraction with the use of forceps or cesarean section during labor than in infants delivered by cesarean section without labor or spontaneous vaginal delivery [18]. The rates of intracranial hemorrhage, however, were low for all modes of delivery. Badawi and colleagues' case-control study investigating the intrapartum causes of neonatal encephalopathy showed that operative vaginal delivery and emergency cesarean section were associated with increased risk for neonatal encephalopathy [19]. Conversely, elective cesarean section was associated with reduced risk for neonatal encephalopathy.

In a study that compared infants born by elective repeat cesarean section to those born vaginally, a statistically significant increase in suspected sepsis was noted in infants delivered vaginally [20]. The increased rate of sepsis evaluation in neonates born to mothers after a trial of vaginal delivery also was seen in a recent study by Signore and coworkers [21].

Regarding nonmaleficence, the increased neonatal respiratory morbidities associated with cesarean deliveries, shown in several studies, should be considered. Transient tachypnea of the newborn (TTN), persistent pulmonary hypertension, and respiratory distress syndrome all have been seen at increased rates in infants born by cesarean section compared with those born vaginally [22–28]. Iatrogenic prematurity, that is the delivery of an infant at less than 37weeks' gestation, may contribute to much of the increased respiratory distress syndrome seen in infants delivered by elective cesarean section. Delivery by cesarean section, however, also is an independent risk factor for the development of respiratory distress syndrome [29]. To avoid iatrogenic prematurity, many physicians recommend delaying cesareans until after the 39th week.

TTN results from delayed clearance of fetal lung fluid [30,31]. Although TTN typically is a benign, self-limited illness that requires minimal intervention, some infants may go on to develop pulmonary hypertension and even to require extracorporeal membrane oxygenation (ECMO) [32–34]. Additionally, in a recent study (published in the *Journal of Pediatrics*), TTN was associated with an increased risk for wheezing syndromes in later childhood [35].

There is an increased risk for stillbirth in infants born to pregnant women given a trial of labor [36]. Neonatal mortality is increased, however, in infants born by cesarean section [21]. Overall perinatal mortality is decreased for planned cesarean deliveries.

Justice

The principle of justice includes considering equitable distribution of available medical resources. Distributive justice often is considered in decision making on a societal level rather than as a principle applied to the care of individual patients. To simply consider the cost of the procedure weighs heavily in favor of vaginal delivery [37]. Allen and colleagues' study examined the costs of hospital care associated with different methods of delivery for nulliparous women. In this cost analysis, the least expensive delivery was spontaneous vaginal delivery. Cesarean delivery in labor was the most costly and significantly more costly than cesarean delivery with no labor.

For a true estimate of the economic impact of CDMR, however, the long-term maternal and neonatal morbidities and the costs associated with these complications must be considered. Druzin and El-Sayed's recent review in *Seminars in Perinatology* asks whether or not CDMR is a wise use of finite resources [38]. They conclude, "promotion of primary cesarean section on request as a standard of care, or as a mandated part of patient counseling for delivery, will result in a highly questionable use of finite resources." Other factors influencing the short-term economic impact of CDMR include increased length of stay, need for intensive care, and cost of neonatal and maternal transport.

The ethics of a randomized clinical trial in elective cesarean delivery

The feasibility of a randomized clinical trial comparing elective cesarean delivery and planned vaginal delivery was discussed in a recent article by Ecker [36].

Many investigators agree that the question of CDMR will not be adequately resolved until a randomized controlled trial is undertaken. The majority of studies published thus far comparing outcomes between cesarean and vaginal deliveries have been retrospective case-control studies. As a result of the limited and often conflicting information gathered from these trials, it is difficult and confusing to counsel patients. Experts vary in their conclusions about these studies, some concluding that CDMR is acceptable and should be an option for all women and others concluding that CDMR is an unacceptable, worrisome practice. As a result of this high degree of uncertainty, it can be argued that equipoise exists and a large-scale randomized clinical trial is ethically appropriate. Nygaard and Cruikshank [39] caution, however, that a randomized controlled trial may be limited in its generalizability to populations outside of the study and may be restricted by the short follow-up inherent in clinical trials. Additionally, it may prove difficult to enroll women willing to be randomized to cesarean delivery versus planned vaginal delivery. Any changes in practice require an improved scientific basis.

The American College of Obstetricians and Gynecologists in its opinion on surgery and patient choice states, "in the absence of significant data on the risks and benefits of cesarean delivery, the burden of proof should fall on those who are advocates for a change in policy in support of elective cesarean delivery (ie, the replacement of a natural process with a major surgical procedure)" [40]. This statement echoes the cry for further research before widespread changes in practice are recommended.

Summary

Cesarean births in the United States are on the rise and a large number of primary cesareans may have been performed on maternal request, without any obstetric or medical indications. This trend may be fueled by concerns about maternal morbidities, especially damage to the pelvic floor. There is a great deal of conflicting evidence concerning maternal and neonatal morbidities associated with cesarean delivery. These limitations must be acknowledged in discussing options with patients and in obtaining informed consent. A randomized trial, although ethically controversial, may help to clarify some of the risks and benefits of elective cesarean delivery. Based on currently available evidence, elective cesarean sections should not be recommended before 39 weeks' gestation or for women who desire several children.

Acknowledgments

Thanks to Kathy Kinlaw, M.Div, for her assistance with preparation of this manuscript.

References

[1] Hamilton BE, Martin JA, Ventura SJ. Births: preliminary data for 2005. Natl Vital Stat Rep 2006;55(11):1–18.

[2] Anonymous. NIH state-of-the-science conference statement on cesarean delivery on maternal request. NIH Consens State Sci Statements 2006;23(1):1–29.

[3] Meikle SF, Steiner CA, Zhang J, et al. A national estimate of the elective primary cesarean delivery rate. Obstet Gynecol 2005;105(4):751–6.

[4] Wax JR, Cartin A, Pinette MG, et al. Patient choice cesarean: an evidence-based review. Obstet Gynecol Surv 2004;59(8):601–16.

[5] Beauchamp TL, Childress JF. Principles of biomedical ethics. 5th edition. New York: Oxford University Press; 2001. p. xi, 454.

[6] Farrell SA, Baskett TF, Farrell KD. The choice of elective cesarean delivery in obstetrics: a voluntary survey of Canadian health care professionals. Int Urogynecol J Pelvic Floor Dysfunct 2005;16(5):378–83.

[7] Minkoff H, Chervenak FA. Elective primary cesarean delivery. N Engl J Med 2003;348(10): 946–50.

[8] Wu JM, Hundley AF, Visco AG. Elective primary cesarean delivery: attitudes of urogynecology and maternal-fetal medicine specialists. Obstet Gynecol 2005;105(2):301–6.

[9] Dietz HP. Pelvic floor trauma following vaginal delivery. Curr Opin Obstet Gynecol 2006; 18(5):528–37.

[10] Hannah ME, Hannah WJ, Hodnett ED, et al. Outcomes at 3 months after planned cesarean vs planned vaginal delivery for breech presentation at term: the international randomized Term Breech Trial. JAMA 2002;287(14):1822–31.

[11] Hannah ME, Whyte H, Hannah WJ, et al. Maternal outcomes at 2 years after planned cesarean section versus planned vaginal birth for breech presentation at term: the international randomized Term Breech Trial. Am J Obstet Gynecol 2004;191(3):917–27.

[12] Rortveit G, Daltveit AK, Hannestad YS, et al. Urinary incontinence after vaginal delivery or cesarean section. N Engl J Med 2003;348(10):900–7.

[13] Borello-France D, Burgio KL, Richter HE, et al. Fecal and urinary incontinence in primiparous women. Obstet Gynecol 2006;108(4):863–72.

[14] Nygaard I. Urinary incontinence: is cesarean delivery protective? Semin Perinatol 2006; 30(5):267–71.

[15] Silver RM, Landon MB, Rouse DJ, et al. Maternal morbidity associated with multiple repeat cesarean deliveriesObstet Gynecol 2006;107(6):1226–32.

[16] Faiz AS, Ananth CV. Etiology and risk factors for placenta previa: an overview and meta-analysis of observational studies. J Matern Fetal Neonatal Med 2003;13(3):175–90.

[17] Visco AG, Viswanathan M, Lohr KN, et al. Cesarean delivery on maternal request: maternal and neonatal outcomes. Obstet Gynecol 2006;108(6):1517–29.

[18] Towner D, Castro MA, Eby-Wilkens E, et al. Effect of mode of delivery in nulliparous women on neonatal intracranial injury [see comment]. N Engl J Med 1999;341(23):1709–14.

[19] Badawi N, Kurinczuk JJ, Keogh JM, et al. Intrapartum risk factors for newborn encephalopathy: the Western Australian case-control study [see comment]. BMJ 1998;317(7172):1554–8.

[20] Hook B, Kiwi R, Amini SB, et al. Neonatal morbidity after elective repeat cesarean section and trial of labor. Pediatrics 1997;100(3 Pt 1):348–53.

[21] Signore C, Hemachandra A, Klebanoff M. Neonatal mortality and morbidity after elective cesarean delivery versus routine expectant management: a decision analysis. Semin Perinatol 2006;30(5):288–95.

[22] Kolas T, Saugstad OD, Daltveit AK, et al. Planned cesarean versus planned vaginal delivery at term: comparison of newborn infant outcomes. Am J Obstet Gynecol 2006;195(6): 1538–43.

[23] Levine EM, Ghai V, Barton JJ, et al. Mode of delivery and risk of respiratory diseases in newborns. Obstet Gynecol 2001;97(3):439–42.

[24] Zanardo V, Simbi AK, Franzoi M, et al. Neonatal respiratory morbidity risk and mode of delivery at term: influence of timing of elective caesarean delivery. Acta Paediatr 2004;93(5): 643–7.

[25] Alderdice F, McCall E, Bailie C, et al. Admission to neonatal intensive care with respiratory morbidity following 'term' elective caesarean section. Ir Med J 2005;98(6):170–2.

[26] Wax JR, Herson V, Carignan E, et al. Contribution of elective delivery to severe respiratory distress at term. Am J Perinatol 2002;19(2):81–6.

[27] van den Berg A, van Elburg RM, van Geijn HP, et al. Neonatal respiratory morbidity following elective caesarean section in term infants. A 5-year retrospective study and a review of the literature [review] [32 refs]. Eur J Obstet Gynecol Reprod Biol 2001;98(1):9–13.

[28] Fogelson NS, Menard MK, Hulsey T, et al. Neonatal impact of elective repeat cesarean delivery at term: a comment on patient choice cesarean delivery. Am J Obstet Gynecol 2005; 192(5):1433–6.

[29] Gerten KA, Coonrod DV, Bay RC, et al. Cesarean delivery and respiratory distress syndrome: does labor make a difference? [see comment] Am J Obstet Gynecol 2005; 193(3 Pt 2):1061–4.

[30] Jain L, Dudell GG. Respiratory transition in infants delivered by cesarean section. Semin Perinatol 2006;30(5):296–304.

[31] Jain L, Eaton DC. Physiology of fetal lung fluid clearance and the effect of labor. Semin Perinatol 2006;30(1):34–43.

[32] Keszler M, Carbone MT, Cox C, et al. Severe respiratory failure after elective repeat cesarean delivery: a potentially preventable condition leading to extracorporeal membrane oxygenation. Pediatrics 1992;89(4 Pt 1):670–2.

[33] Heritage CK, Cunningham MD. Association of elective repeat cesarean delivery and persistent pulmonary hypertension of the newborn. Am J Obstet Gynecol 1985;152(6 Pt 1):627–9.

[34] Hernandez-Diaz S, Van Marter LJ, Werler MM, et al. Risk factors for persistent pulmonary hypertension of the newborn. Pediatrics 2007;120(2):e272–82.

[35] Liem JJ, Huq SI, Ekuma O, et al. Transient tachypnea of the newborn may be an early clinical manifestation of wheezing symptoms. J Pediatr 2007;151(1):29–33.
[36] Ecker JL. Once a pregnancy, always a cesarean? Rationale and feasibility of a randomized controlled trial. Am J Obstet Gynecol 2004;190(2):314–8.
[37] Allen VM, O'Connell CM, Baskett TF. Cumulative economic implications of initial method of delivery. Obstet Gynecol 2006;108(3 Pt 1):549–55.
[38] Druzin ML, El-Sayed YY. Cesarean delivery on maternal request: wise use of finite resources? A view from the trenches. Semin Perinatol 2006;30(5):305–8.
[39] Nygaard I, Cruikshank DP. Should all women be offered elective cesarean delivery? Obstet Gynecol 2003;102(2):217–9.
[40] ACOG Committee Opinion. Surgery and patient choice: the ethics of decision makingObstet Gynecol 2003;102(5 Pt 1):1101–6.

**ELSEVIER
SAUNDERS**

CLINICS IN
PERINATOLOGY

Clin Perinatol 35 (2008) 463–467

Index

Note: Page numbers of article titles are in **boldface** type.